HYPERBARIC OXYGEN THERAPY

Richard A. Neubauer, MD
Morton Walker, DPM

A DR. MORTON WALKER HEALTH BOOK

AVERY
a member of Penguin Putnam Inc.

The therapeutic procedures in this book are based on the training, personal experiences, and research of the authors. Because each person and situation is unique, the authors and publisher urge the reader to check with a qualified health professional before using any procedure when there is any question regarding the presence or treatment of any abnormal health condition.

The publisher does not advocate the use of any particular treatment, but believes the information presented in this book should be available to the public.

Because there is always some risk involved, the author and publisher are not responsible for any adverse effects or consequences resulting from the use of any of the suggestions, preparations, or procedures described in this book. Please do not use the book if you are unwilling to assume the risk. Feel free to consult with a physician or other qualified health professional. It is a sign of wisdom, not cowardice, to seek a second or third opinion.

Cover Design:
William Gonzalez and
   Rudy Shur
Typesetters: Al Berotti and
   Elaine V. McCaw
In-House Editor: Lisa James

Avery
a member of
Penguin Putnam Inc.
375 Hudson Street
New York, NY 10014
www.penguinputnam.com

Library of Congress Cataloging-in Publication Data

Neubauer, Richard A.
   Hyperbaric oxygen therapy : using HBO therapy to increase
circulation, repair damaged tissue, fight infection, save limbs,
relieve pain, and more / by Richard Neubauer and Morton Walker.
     p.   cm.
   Includes bibliographical references and index.
   ISBN 0-89529-759-0
   1. Hyperbaric oxygenation—Popular works. I. Walker, Morton.
II. Title.
RM666.083N48   1998
615.8'36—dc21   97-30980
                                            CIP

Printed in the United States of America

10 9 8 7 6 5 4

Contents

From Morton Walker, D.P.M.
to
Joan Walker,
my loving wife and best friend for these past forty-six years

From Richard A. Neubauer, M.D.
to
Edgar End, M.D. (1910–1983),
the visionary genius of hyperbaric/underwater medicine

Acknowledgments

From Dr. Richard Neubauer: I wish to express my deepest thanks and gratitude to everyone who contributed their time, energy, and talent to this book—it would have not been possible without them. First, I wish to thank my professional colleagues for generously sharing their knowledge and insight: Thomas Bozzuto, M.D.; William Fife, Ph.D.; Harry Goldsmith, M.D.; Sheldon Gottlieb, Ph.D.; William S. Maxfield Sr., M.D.; Barbara Nelson, M.D.; Michelle Reillo, B.S.N., R.N.; and David Youngblood, M.D. I also wish to thank the staff of the Ocean Hyperbaric Center, especially my daughter, Ginger, for their dedication and hard work. Finally, I wish to thank my wife, Winnie, for all her love and support.

Foreword

Adopting it as a therapeutic agent from deep sea commercial diving and from navies around the world, the medical profession has been administering oxygen under pressure to patients. Until now, there has been very little written on the subject for the general public. But that situation finally has changed. *Hyperbaric Oxygen Therapy*, authored by Richard A. Neubauer, M.D. and Morton Walker, D.P.M., offers easy-to-understand information for the medical consumer.

Hyperbaric Oxygen Therapy is about the highly effective, 300-year-old treatment modality called hyperbaric oxygenation. It is a medical tool of great potential importance that I personally receive regularly as the means of overcoming residual stroke symptoms. Yes, at this very time, I am recovering from a stroke caused by a clot that blocked blood flow in the brain. A region of my brain, perhaps one-tenth of an inch in size, has ceased to function due to lack of oxygen. Temporarily? Permanently? The fact that some people make a spontaneous recovery from stroke shows that its effects can be self-healing, but there's a strong possibility that my healing will be accelerated by oxygen diffusing in from some nearby capillary that hasn't been affected by the stroke. Whatever healing occurs will happen faster and more extensively as a result of hyperbaric oxygenation. So, I am presently undergoing a daily two-hour treatment in a hyperbaric chamber, and I'm clearly aware of the recovery of my memories.

Possibly the most important application of hyperbaric oxygen therapy (HBOT), the most natural of medications, is being explored by Dr. Richard Neubauer in the recovery of patients from stroke, multiple sclerosis, coma, and other brain problems.

HBOT is a method of restoring wellness by utilization of the principles pertaining to gases and their physiological effects. These effects can reverse pathological states in which the fact that too little oxygen is reaching the cells (a condition called hypoxia) is a component.

The underlying principle is simple. Oxygen is delivered to tissues and cells by being temporarily incorporated into the hemoglobin contained within our red blood cells. Under normal conditions, hemoglobin is almost 100 percent saturated with oxygen when exposed in our lungs to the atmosphere (which is one-fifth oxygen). It delivers the oxygen to cells with which the blood comes into contact. Hyperbaric oxygen is of use if some tissues or cells are deprived of their contact with blood and obtain either no oxygen or too little oxygen.

When HBOT is used, the oxygen molecules are up to ten times more abundant than they are in air. Hardly any more oxygen is to be imparted to the hemoglobin. But the bulk of the blood, called blood plasma, which is essentially water, dissolves some oxygen. The blood plasma parts with its oxygen contents much more easily than hemoglobin does. If an oxygen-deficient cell is not in contact with a blood capillary but is within a short range of such a capillary (one-hundredth of an inch or a little more), then the oxygen can diffuse from the capillary to the cell and relieve the cell's oxygen hunger, or hypoxia.

Research on hyperbaric oxygen has proven conclusively that relatively low-level deliveries of oxygen to a patient has no ill effects. There are proven indications that the effects can be positive and decisive.

Animal studies show strongly that healing of severe wounds is accelerated by at least 30 percent through treatment with hyperbaric oxygen. Indeed, healing is very frequently slowed down by a scarcity of oxygen. HBOT helps in the formation of new blood vessels. It would seem plausible that if in our hospitals severe surgery would be followed by the use of hyperbaric oxygen, healing would be accelerated by 30 percent. This alone would result in the saving of billions of dollars, not to even mention the reduction in human suffering.

Unlike some other fields of medicine, the clinical aspects of diving hyperbarics (gas pressure above one atmosphere) were developed by military personnel, whereas clinical HBOT used for medical consumers was developed primarily by civilian health professionals. Dr. Richard Neubauer, an internist by training, is one of those health practitioners who has pioneered the use of pure oxygen under elevated pressure for the treatment of brain pathologies.

Recognizing the great value of hyperbaric oxygenation after receiving the therapy himself, Dr. Morton Walker enthusiastically joins with Dr. Neubauer to bring the message of this treatment to a needy readership. *Hyperbaric Oxygen Therapy* is the result of this collaboration.

For the past three decades, hyperbaric oxygen has been applied worldwide. Unfortunately, its use has been much more restricted in the United States than in other countries. However, I hope that broad distribution of this book will encourage the increased usage of HBOT. Many lives, limbs, and minds could be saved by introducing HBOT into all hospitals and using the treatment after every major surgical operation. By means of HBOT, suffering would be reduced. There is no question in my mind that more clinical and laboratory research concerning hyperbaric oxygen, and a better public understanding of the effects and possibilities of this treatment, could lead to considerable improvement in the health of millions.

The intellectual stimulation caused by, and the practical application of, the ideas contained within *Hyperbaric Oxy-*

gen Therapy are factors that should bring about the mandatory expansive use of HBOT. Because this book is written by two experts, with the consultant being a renowned hyperbaricist with an internationally acclaimed reputation, the reader readily learns about the clinical applications of hyperbaric oxygen.

This book is clearly written, concise but comprehensive, explicit in its details, founded on good science, and timely in its presentation of HBOT. Case histories cited, authorities quoted, research literature included—all contribute to a well-rounded and enjoyable piece of writing on what can be a difficult subject.

I am ever so happy to write this foreword as a small contribution toward spreading information about hyperbaric oxygenation. People everywhere deserve this opportunity to be informed about a remarkable therapy that too long has been held back from more extensive use.

Edward Teller, Ph.D.
Director Emeritus, Lawrence Livermore National Laboratory
University Professor Emeritus, University of California
University of California Research Fellow,
Hoover Institution of War, Revolution, and Peace,
Stanford University

Preface

On June 9, 1980, as two police officers patrolled the north-west area of the San Fernando Valley in California, they heard screams of terror. They turned into a street and saw a man running wildly in circles while his upper body and head were encased in blue flames. The officers jumped from their patrol car, wrestled the burning man down, and rolled him in the grass to extinguish the fire. This severely burnt person turned out to be actor and comedian Richard Pryor, who had accidentally set himself ablaze. The officers rushed him to Sherman Oaks Community Hospital and into the care of plastic surgeon Dr. Richard Grossman.

Seriously burned people are at risk of death from many sources simultaneously: shock, loss of body fluids, dysfunction of the kidneys and gastrointestinal tract, lung damage resulting from smoke inhalation, blood poisoning due to various bacteria, and strain on heart function from the terror and pain of the experience. Pryor had all of these things, and his chances of survival were less than 50 percent. Third-degree burns covered his face, ears, chest, arms, and abdomen. If he lived, scarring would likely leave the actor horribly deformed.

Yet, for years afterwards, Richard Pryor performed in front of motion picture and television cameras, on stage, and in nightclubs. Even after contracting multiple sclerosis, the actor continued working. One of the main reasons for this remarkable recovery is that Dr. Grossman uses hyperbaric oxygen therapy (HBOT) in his treatment of burns and skin grafts. During the summer of 1980, at least once every day, Pryor entered the hospital's hyperbaric chamber for an hour at a time. Later, the chamber was used to heal the unburned portions of the actor's body that became donor sites from which his plastic surgeon took skin for grafts. Pryor continued taking HBOT even after his burns and grafts had healed.

That Richard Pryor should benefit from the use of hyperbaric oxygen did not surprise his doctor. In 1978, Dr. Grossman had presented his highly successful clinical experience with HBOT to a group of his colleagues, experience that included 800 patients and covered six years. He reported a sharp reduction in all complications associated with severely burned patients compared with burn patients who were not treated with hyperbaric oxygen. (See Chapter 7 for more information on Dr. Grossman's work.)

Can hyperbaric oxygen help you or someone you love? This book explains what HBOT is and how it can be used in the treatment of a number of different diseases and conditions. In essence, HBOT involves the use of pure oxygen at higher-than-atmospheric pressure to help overcome diseases associated with a lack of oxygen in the tissues. (Normal atmospheric pressure simply isn't strong enough to force the proper amount of oxygen into the body under such conditions.) While not yet a routine part of conventional medical treatment, HBOT may be considered as a form of complementary medicine—a treatment that can be used in addition to the many conventional means of restoring patients to health. No other general book on this subject exists for the medical consumer.

HBOT cannot help all patients, nor is it successful in treating all conditions. In accordance with the best principles of the self-correcting workings of science, some of the diseases for which hyperbaric oxygen was originally thought to be useful have proven themselves unresponsive to HBOT. For example, this treatment is no longer considered beneficial by doctors in the United States for use in routine heart surgery, as an adjunct to cancer chemotherapy, or in the reversal of senility.

American doctors accept HBOT for use in wound healing, bone infection, carbon monoxide intoxication, and air emboli, or air bubbles in the bloodstream due to decompression sickness (see Chapter 1), open-heart surgery, and other sources. But it has been discovered that HBOT can also be used for conditions such as coma resulting from head injuries, bruising of the spinal cord, stroke, and neurological disorders such as multiple sclerosis. These additional applications have yet to be recognized by the medical establishment in this country, although they have been accepted in other countries.

Scientific evidence indicates strongly that oxygen administered under appropriate pressure is a remarkable and versatile treatment. However, it is overlooked, due in part to a lack of public and medical-community information on the subject. In this book, we aim to correct that long-standing omission. HBOT has too much potential as a life-improving treatment for too many people to allow its continued neglect. We believe there are many people who can be aided by HBOT.

Why is there such a lack of knowledge among doctors about HBOT? There are several reasons. One is that many doctors do not realize that HBOT can force oxygen into the body's tissues. Most diseases affect an area's microcirculation, the circulation through the tiny capillaries that connect arteries to veins. The damage results in a loss of oxygen to tissue. The use of normal-pressure oxygen forces oxygen into the red blood cells, which usually carry oxygen. But the administration of high-pressure oxygen forces oxygen into the blood plasma, the liquid part of the bloodstream, which normally doesn't carry the life-giving gas. By forcing oxygen into the blood plasma, and not just the red blood cells, HBOT can help bring oxygen to areas of the body in which circulation has been impaired, especially since oxygen under pressure not only dissolves in the plasma but in all the body's fluids, such as the lymph and the fluid surrounding the brain and spine, as well as in bone marrow.

Most doctors are also not familiar with the basic science regarding HBOT. Many seem to regard pressurized oxygen as being chemically different from the normal-pressure oxygen, which it isn't. Some are not familiar with the basic gas laws of physics, since this is a topic not covered in medical school. And a few seem to believe that the healing promoted by hyperbaric oxygen is only temporary. It's not. Doctors are not familiar with HBOT, and most do not wish to look into the matter. They are reluctant to investigate new therapies.

Another factor is that oxygen under pressure is not a manufactured drug, whereas medical practice in nearly all industrialized countries is dominated by the drug industry. This means there is no commercial promotion for HBOT as there is for pharmaceuticals.

Finally, hyperbaric oxygenation falls into a class of therapy similar to that developed by the American-born Sir Hiram Maxim. Sir Hiram invented the machine gun, which revolutionized warfare and for which he won fame, fortune, and knighthood. Sir Hiram, a chronic sufferer of bronchitis, also invented a relatively simple steam inhaler, which he found exceedingly helpful in treating his disease. (Thousands of homes today have small portable humidifiers built according to the principles that Sir Hiram developed.) He decided to market his helpful new invention and was promptly met with a storm of accusations. Both the organized medical establishment and the media of his time claimed that he was, in his words, "prostituting my talents on quack nostrums." Shortly before his death, Sir Hiram wryly commented: "From the foregoing it will be seen that it is a very creditable thing to invent a killing machine, and nothing less than a disgrace to invent an apparatus to prevent human suffering."

Like Sir Hiram's steam inhaler, HBOT has faced a difficult time in becoming accepted by organized medicine. Even with over 30,000 scientific studies on HBOT published in medical journals, diving medicine journals, and clinical journals of the other health care disciplines, there has been strong resistance from those representing the Western medical establishment.

It must fall, then, to the medical consumer to become well educated about HBOT's merits, and to demand access to this treatment. That is what will need to happen before HBOT is widely used, and that is why we have written this book—for your edification and action.

CHAPTER 1

Oxygen
Under Pressure—
Hyperbaric Oxygen Therapy

In Georgia, 76-year-old Raymond N. suffers an apparent stroke that leaves him with dizziness, confusion, and weakness on his right side. Brain scans indicate that the damage probably comes from a reduction in blood flow through an artery in the middle of his brain. Within six hours, Raymond receives hyperbaric oxygen therapy. A scan taken after one session shows a marked improvement in the amount of oxygen reaching the affected areas of Raymond's brain. After ten sessions, he shows complete improvement.

In Texas, 38-year-old Florence A., a busy attorney and mother of three, is suddenly struck with symptoms of multiple sclerosis. She seeks out every type of treatment available and finds that many of the treatments do more harm than good. Within two years, she is blind and wheelchair-bound. She then begins a series of sessions in a hyperbaric oxygen chamber. "From being totally blind, I could see again in order to read a novel or a spreadsheet," she says. She's also able to walk on her own. Florence resumes the life she had known before her illness, and makes time for periodic follow-up sessions in the chamber.

In Texas, 22-year-old Laura C., a sculptor, severs her left hand while working at a band saw. She is taken to a hospital, where surgeons re-attach her hand. As time goes on, she needs three additional surgeries, as well as physical therapy. Throughout the recovery process, Laura is treated with HBOT. While she still experiences some problems with sensation, the hand functions normally. She can play the piano and use a typewriter—and sculpt.

What do people who suffer strokes, multiple sclerosis attacks, and severed limbs have in common? All can be helped by hyperbaric oxygen therapy (HBOT). Patients who receive HBOT breathe pure oxygen—the gas that keeps us alive—while in pressurized chambers, which forces the oxygen into the body's tissues. While HBOT is certainly no miracle cure, the extra oxygen it provides can help people with numerous conditions live healthier, longer, and more comfortable lives.

HBOT causes no pain or discomfort, and carries a very low risk of side effects. Around the world, hundreds of thousands of people have spent time in hyperbaric oxygen chambers.

There is also a considerable amount of research that supports the use of HBOT. For example, in one study, the cases of 50 patients who had suffered acute stroke were analyzed. Half of them had received HBOT, while the other half had received conventional therapy. The study showed that the average hospital stay for the patients given HBOT was substantially shorter than for the other patients. There was only one death in the HBOT group, compared with three deaths in the conventional therapy group. All of the surviving HBOT patients returned home to their families, while 40 percent of those not treated with HBOT required nursing home care.

In this chapter, we will see how HBOT works, what conditions it can be used to treat, and how it was developed. We will then look at HBOT's excellent safety record and why this therapy is not used as much as it could be.

WHAT IS HYPERBARIC OXYGEN THERAPY?

HBOT is a method of administering pure oxygen at greater than atmospheric pressure to a patient in order to improve or correct certain conditions. (For an explanation of what atmospheric pressure is, see "The Language of HBOT and of Research" on page 7.) The procedure is quite comfortable and may even occasionally leave the patient with a sense of well-being.

Most often, HBOT is given as a one- to two-hour treatment in a specially designed, sealed chamber. The chamber can vary in size from a small, one-person monoplace unit to a large, multiplace unit capable of housing an entire surgical team. There are even portable chambers that can be brought to the scene of an emergency.

In the monoplace chamber (see Figure 1.1), the entire chamber is pressurized with oxygen. In the multiplace chamber (see Figure 1.2), the patient receives oxygen by either hood or mask while the chamber is pressurized with normal air. While in the chamber, the patient can watch television, listen to music, or simply rest. The monoplace chamber is easier to use in an emergency because it requires less preparation and fewer operators. (See Appendix A for information on contacting hyperbaric oxygen facilities.)

Why does HBOT help speed the healing process? Nature has dictated that healing cannot take place without appropriate oxygen levels in the body's tissues. In many cases, such as those involving circulatory problems and strokes, adequate oxygen can't reach the damaged area, and the body's natural healing process fails to function properly. Breathing oxygen under pressure can, at times, overcome this oxygen starvation.

Why is oxygen so important? Oxygen is a colorless, odorless gas that makes up about 21 percent of the atmosphere. It is essential to life for two reasons. First, oxygen is one of the body's basic building blocks. All of the body's major components—water, protein, carbohydrate, and fat—contain oxygen. Second, oxygen helps bring about certain chemical reactions within the body that result in energy production. Energy is needed for functions such as circulation, respiration, and digestion. Energy is also used to maintain a constant body temperature.

If the body is totally deprived of oxygen, death results within minutes. A diminished supply of oxygen causes

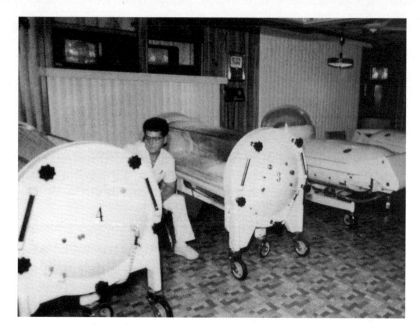

Figure 1.1. Monoplace Chamber

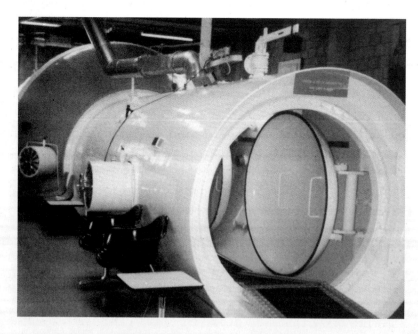

Figure 1.2. Multiplace Chamber

multiple symptoms, some of which are mental disturbances, shortness of breath and rapid pulse, a fall in blood pressure, and *cyanosis*, a blueness of the skin and mucous membranes. There is a marked reduction in all bodily functions. This condition is known as *hypoxia*, or under-oxygenation of the tissues.

How does HBOT force more oxygen into the bloodstream, and therefore into the tissues? Blood is made up of three main components: white cells that fight infection, red cells that carry oxygen, and plasma, the fluid that carries both kinds of cells throughout the body. Under normal circumstances, only the red blood cells carry oxygen. But because HBOT forces oxygen into the body under pressure, oxygen dissolves into all of the body's fluids, including the plasma, the lymph, the cerebrospinal fluid surrounding the brain and spinal cord. These fluids can carry the extra oxygen even to areas where circulation is poor or blocked, either by trickling past blockages or by seeping into the affected area.

This extra oxygen helps the healing process. It enhances the white blood cells' ability to fight infection. It can promote the development of new capillaries, the tiny blood vessels that connect arteries to veins. It helps the body build new connective tissue. And it helps the organs function the way that they should.

For years, conventional medicine thought of HBOT only as a treatment for decompression sickness and air embolism (see page 9). However, the use of HBOT is becoming increasingly common in general medical practice as more doctors become acquainted with its applications. Doctors now realize there are other uses for HBOT,[1-4] including treatment of nonhealing wounds, carbon monoxide poisoning, various infections, damage caused by radiation treatments, and all types of diving accidents. But it can be used to treat dozens of additional diseases and conditions, including near-drowning, near-hanging, and near-electrocution; brain and nerve disorders; cardiovascular disorders; and some digestive system disorders. (See Appendix B for

a list of conditions that have been treated with HBOT.)
The conditions covered in this book are:

• Stroke (see Chapter 2)

• Brain and spinal cord injuries; migraine headaches; and
  sensory problems, such as tinnitus and macular degeneration (see Chapter 3)

• Multiple sclerosis (see Chapter 4)

• Difficult wounds (see Chapter 5)

• Infections (see Chapter 6)

• Burns (see Chapter 7)

• Bone disorders, such as infections, inflammations, and
  fractures that won't heal (see Chapter 8)

• Complications, such as those that result from radiation
  treatment and cosmetic surgery (see Chapter 9)

• Poisoning, including carbon monoxide poisoning (see
  Chapter 10)

• Circulatory problems (see Chapter 11)

• AIDS (see Chapter 12)

It is important to realize that, in most cases, HBOT is
not a primary treatment. That means that HBOT is best
used when combined with other treatments, such as physical therapy, drugs, or surgery. Among the few conditions
for which HBOT is a primary treatment are diving accidents, gas gangrene, and carbon monoxide poisoning.

THE HISTORY OF HBOT

For more than three hundred years, people have been
breathing pressurized air for its therapeutic effect.[5,6] A
British physician named Henshaw is believed to have been
the first, in 1664, to use compressed air in a specially
equipped room called a domicilium. Henshaw believed
that breathing vigorously inside the domicilium improved
both digestion and respiration.

The Language of HBOT and of Research

It is easier to understand the concepts behind HBOT if you understand some basic terms. One of these terms is *atmospheric pressure*. The air around us exerts pressure because it has weight, that is, it is being pulled towards the Earth's center by gravity. Atmospheric pressure decreases as one climbs above sea level because the column of air over one's head weighs less the higher one goes. As one dives below the surface of the ocean, pressure increases because the column of water above one's head weighs more the deeper one goes. The increase is rapid because water weighs more than air. This water pressure is called *hydrostatic pressure*. Total pressure is the hydrostatic pressure plus the atmospheric pressure, since the atmosphere also exerts its weight on the surface of the water. This total pressure is called absolute atmospheric pressure, or *atmospheres absolute*.

We can measure pressure in a number of ways. One unit of measurement is *pounds per square inch (psi)*. For example, tire pressure is measured in psi. However, when discussing high pressure, or *hyperbaric*, oxygen, the measurement unit used is the atmospheres absolute. One atmospheres absolute is the average atmospheric pressure exerted at sea level, or 14.7 psi. Pressures greater than 1.0 atmospheres absolute are expressed in terms of additional atmospheres absolute or fractions of atmospheres absolute. For example, a doctor may prescribe one hour of HBOT at 1.5 atmospheres absolute, or one and a half times the average sea-level pressure. A *dose* of oxygen depends on how much pressure is used, how long the pressure is maintained, and the frequency and total number of treatments.

There are several basic types of medical studies. *Case studies* are studies that analyze what happens when a treatment is administered to actual patients. These studies reveal whether or not a treatment works, what patients it works best on, and so forth.

Placebo-controlled, double-blind studies compare the treatment being tested with a control. This gives the doctors conducting the test something against which to measure the treatment's effectiveness. People in the control group are given an inert substance called a placebo. Double-blind means that neither the doctors nor the participants know which participants are controls and which are actual test subjects. This prevents false positive results caused by psychological effects, and guards against special treatment of either the volunteers or the data by the investigators. At times, double-blind studies jeopardize certain patients, and may therefore be inappropriate in certain situations.

Crossover studies are those in which a patient receives either the placebo or the test treatment for the first part of the study, and then switches to the other substance for the second part. This allows the researcher to find out whether the test treatment works or not, without threatening the health of the patient. In effect, the patient serves as his or her own control.

Most patients treated with HBOT have been unsuccessfully exposed to every other available treatment before HBOT is finally used. The cases of such patients represent *longitudinal studies*, that is, studies in which patients essentially serve as their own controls because HBOT is the last in a series of documented treatments. Thus, these cases cannot be dismissed as anecdotal evidence, or evidence based merely on the patient's subjective reaction to HBOT.

The effects of pressure on the body were most noticed by divers because of the greater pressures encountered underwater (see "The Language of HBOT and of Research"). Therefore, HBOT developed largely in response to the problems experienced by divers.

Two of the most serious problems divers face are air embolism and decompression sickness, also referred to as "the bends." Divers breathe compressed air, which is 79 percent nitrogen. When a diver descends, both oxygen and nitrogen from the compressed air dissolve in the blood. The longer the diver stays at an increased pressure, the more gas is dissolved. As long as the diver stays at this increased pressure, the gas remains dissolved, and the diver is in no danger.

If the diver ascends while holding his or her breath, the lungs can overexpand and tear internally, forcing bubbles of gas into the bloodstream. These bubbles can block off blood flow to various parts of the diver's body, especially the brain, which can result in severe tissue damage or even death. Such a bubble is known as an *air embolism*.

Bubbles can form even if the diver breathes correctly. This occurs in situations where large quantities of dissolved gas are present in the body and the diver ascends too quickly (that is, faster than the gas can diffuse from the blood into the lungs for safe elimination). This type of gas-bubble disease is termed *decompression sickness*, or "the bends" (so-called because the knee joints are frequently involved, causing the person to bend forward as he or she walks).

The only way to treat air embolism and decompression sickness is to place the diver in a hyperbaric chamber, which forces the gas bubbles safely back into solution within the body. That allows the gas to be removed from the body via the lungs during a slow, controlled chamber decompression.

A variety of experiments were conducted by English, French, and Dutch researchers using various types of diving apparatus in the eighteenth and nineteenth centuries. But the practical use of pressurized oxygen in commercial and military diving didn't start until 1935. Eventually, navies around the world recognized that breathing oxygen in chambers under elevated atmospheric pressure helped ensure the safety of decompressing divers. After studies were done, suggestions were made as to the appropriate use of pressurized oxygen in the treatment of decompression sickness.[7] As a result, during the 1940s, oxygen was incorporated into standard decompression treatment tables devised by the United States Navy. Studies were also done during World War II on the role of oxygen in high-altitude sickness.

The use of oxygen in the treatment of decompression sickness contributed to the scientific foundation for the application of HBOT in the treatment of other conditions.[8,9] There have been significant improvements in the use of HBOT. Moreover, many claims were made, especially in the 1960s, for its efficacy in reversing certain conditions, such as senility and hair loss. Most of these claims have not withstood scientific scrutiny. But a growing number of conditions have been found to respond to hyperbaric oxygen through both double-blind crossover studies and case studies.

THE SAFETY OF HBOT

It is generally accepted that HBOT is quite safe. HBOT provides extra oxygen with virtually no side effects. The only possible short-term discomfort one might feel is minor ear or sinus pressure, similar to that experienced when ascending or descending in an airplane. HBOT should not be used when there is air in the chest cavity surrounding the lung, a condition called pneumothorax, or when a bubble on the lung itself is likely to rupture. These are fairly rare occurrences. However, it is a good idea for most patients to have a chest examination or chest x-ray before undergoing HBOT.

Still, like any other treatment, HBOT is not without potential problems. Some of these problems are more technical than biological, and have to do with oxygen's chemical nature. A room with high levels of oxygen can fuel fire and explosion. Therefore, flames and electric sparks must be avoided when oxygen is being given.

Hyperbaric oxygen chambers are carefully designed to prevent fire and other dangers. There have been accidents involving such chambers, but they have been very rare, and have generally resulted from errors made by inexperienced technicians. Hyperbaric chambers are manufactured and installed under strictly controlled conditions.

It must also be kept in mind that when oxygen is administered under pressure, it can have a toxic effect if used improperly. This effect appears as seizures that disappear immediately upon reduction of the pressure. It has occasionally been observed at pressures below 3.0 atmospheres absolute, and is virtually unreported at pressures below 2.0 atmospheres absolute. In addition, prolonged administration of HBOT, as in some diving applications, may produce lung irritation.

WHY HBOT IS NOT USED MORE OFTEN

If HBOT is accepted to be a safe treatment, why aren't more doctors prescribing it? We go into this subject in a little more detail in the Conclusion, but basically, most doctors are not yet familiar with hyperbarics. Also, the use of HBOT involves the expense of installing hyperbaric chambers and hiring the technical staff to run them. Another reason is that HBOT is not yet a fully established subject in medical schools. In the United States, only forty-six medical schools teach hyperbaric medicine or have hyperbaric chambers, compared with all medical schools in Italy. Thus, medical students often do not learn about hyperbarics. Practicing doctors don't learn about HBOT because much of their continuing education comes from the pharmaceutical industry, which naturally has no interest in informing doctors about a product it does not sell. Furthermore, it is characteristic of the medical establishment, as with any establishment, to be disposed toward preserving the existing order. If a doctor should become interested in HBOT, he or she must spend a considerable amount of time and effort to search the medical literature for information about this subject.

Unfortunately, disagreements between doctors about the merits of HBOT often have considerable consequences for patients. Either treatment can be denied outright, or insurance carriers will not pay for it. For example, a young Illinois man suffered brain damage after a near-hanging, the result of a suicide attempt. His parents studied various forms of therapy, and decided that HBOT might be able to help their son (see Chapter 3). But the local hospital would not treat the young man in their hyperbaric center because the hospital's doctors didn't believe that HBOT provides any benefits for brain-injured patients.[10] The patient's parents finally took him to an HBOT facility in Florida, and his condition improved after hyperbaric oxygenation treatment.

In another case, a Michigan teenager lapsed into a coma after being struck by lightning. He came out of the coma five months later with severe brain damage. He received dozens of different forms of treatment, but made the greatest progress while receiving HBOT out of state. However, halfway through the course of treatment, the young man's insurance carrier stopped paying, and the young man's parents had to take him home. Unfortunately, the doctors who operated hyperbaric chambers in Wisconsin, Michigan, and Illinois wouldn't treat him, since they didn't believe HBOT to be of any use in treating neurological disorders.

In this chapter, we've taken a general look at HBOT—at what it is, at how it was developed, and at its excellent safety record. In the next chapter, we'll see how hyperbaric oxygen can help improve the lives of stroke patients.

CHAPTER 2

Using HBOT
to Treat Stroke

In Alabama, 58-year-old Larry H., a railroad dispatcher, suffers a stroke. He is bedridden and unresponsive, and the Veterans Administration has classified Larry as being beyond rehabilitation. His wife, Judy, is told that his condition will continue to worsen. Physical therapy does not help. Eventually, Judy hears about HBOT, and takes Larry to Dr. Neubauer's facility in Florida. "After the fourteenth hyperbaric treatment, he amazed us all," Judy says. "[He] spoke words, turned himself over in bed, became progressively active during the day, and actually participated in his physical therapy sessions." He is able to return home, where he and Judy find a nearby hyperbaric facility so that Larry can take follow-up treatments. There is considerable improvement in Larry's ability to participate in the activities of daily living, although Larry does not make a full recovery.

Today, stroke outranks head injury as the leading cause of neurologic disability in the industrialized West. In fact, stroke is the third most frequent cause of death in the United States and the major cause of disability among Americans. One third of those who suffer a stroke do not survive the initial attack, and another third enter nursing homes. Only one third improve, and many of these patients are left with disabilities that hinder their capacity to resume their prestroke lives. Stroke care in the United States costs more than $30 billion a year.

HBOT cannot help all stroke patients, but it does offer some patients and their families new hope. In this chapter, we'll first see why stroke occurs, what symptoms it produces, and what kind of damage it causes. We'll then see how HBOT can revive brain cells surrounding the stroke-affected area, and how a sophisticated body-imaging system called SPECT allows doctors to monitor this revival. (See Appendix A for information on contacting hyperbaric oxygen facilities.)

WHAT IS A STROKE?

Packed within the soft mass of the brain are more than 10 billion interconnected nerve cells, called *neurons*. Though the brain is protected against danger from without by the skull, danger can lurk from within in the form of a blockage or rupture in one or more of the brain's thousands of blood vessels.

Stroke—also called cerebrovascular accident (CVA)—refers to the loss of functioning brain tissue caused by circulation problems within the brain. These circulation problems cut off the brain's supply of blood, and therefore its supply of oxygen. Without oxygen, neurons begin to die. The disabilities that result depend upon what area of the brain has been affected. They include persistent paralysis on one side of the body, and spasticity, or rigid muscles. This damage to the brain can reduce mobility, speech, and swallowing ability, and can result in mental difficulties, including memory loss and personality changes.[1]

A cutoff of blood circulation can occur for one of three reasons. The first is *ischemia*, or lack of blood flow caused by the narrowing or blockage of an artery. Ischemic thrombotic strokes may result from atherosclerosis, commonly called hardening of the arteries, in which plaques of cholesterol and other substances build up on the artery walls. Ischemic thrombotic strokes injure a specific area of the brain supplied by a particular blood vessel and, in so doing, cause a specific loss of function.

A second, related reason a stroke may occur is the development of *emboli*. These are blood clots that sometimes block an artery and cut off blood flow. Clots may travel to the brain via the heart from distant sources, such as the legs, in the uncommon event that a hole exists in the wall between the heart's right and left sides. Emboli can be, but are not always, the cause of ischemic strokes.

The third reason a stroke may occur is *cerebral hemorrhage*. This means there is bleeding within the brain. Massive hemorrhage can destroy large areas on one or both sides of the brain, causing rapid loss of consciousness followed by death. High blood pressure or blood vessel abnormalities can bring on a cerebral hemorrhage. This type of stroke has the highest death rate.

The main warning sign of an impending stroke is the occurrence of *transient ischemic attacks* (TIA). A TIA is a miniature or temporary stroke occurring in a localized area of the brain that lasts from a few minutes to a few hours. Despite its temporary nature, a TIA can cause major problems depending on what area of the brain is affected. A TIA may be produced by a blocked blood vessel, a blood clot, or a buildup of blood fats, but is most often due to a spasm of the blood vessel. It is estimated that approximately thirty-five of every one hundred persons who experience a TIA will suffer a lethal or incapacitating stroke within five years.

No matter what causes a stroke, the result is a localized area of decay in the brain called an *infarct*. In some cases, the tissue within an infarct may wither and create small holes, called *lacunas*. Over the years, the development of lacunas can riddle the brain, causing dementia similar to that seen in Alzheimer's disease. However, it is important to remember that dementia caused by a stroke is not the same thing as that caused by Alzheimer's disease, although they cause the same effects. The brain degeneration seen in Alzheimer's has nothing to do with the circulatory system, and therefore cannot be reversed by the use of HBOT.

Whether or not a patient can recover from a stroke depends upon several factors. One factor is the extent and size of the damaged area. The injured site is like an atom bomb blast, with a central core of irreparably damaged tissue surrounded by an area that is not so heavily damaged. The farther a section of the brain is from the central core, the less likely it is to be impaired.

Between the damaged tissue and the unaffected, normal brain is another zone referred to as the *penumbra*. This exceedingly important area is another factor in determining how much of a recovery the patient can make. That is because the penumbra contains so-called "dormant," or "idling," neurons, brain cells that are nonfunctional but intact. If these cells can be awakened, the patient has a good chance of recovering at least some function. The condition, volume, and location of the penumbra are important considerations.

Another factor in the patient's ability to recover from a stroke is the brain's ability to reorganize itself. In this respect, the stroke-affected brain can be compared to a finished jigsaw puzzle that is broken up, placed in a box, and shaken. If the pieces can be sorted out and reassembled, the picture can be recreated. Likewise, if the brain can at least partially sort out the undamaged cells and reorganize them, the patient can regain at least partial function. Sometimes, one part of the brain can take over the function of another part of the brain. This ability to switch functions is called *plasticity*.

Acute stroke occurs in several main phases. The first is called the *ischemic cascade*. In this phase, which doctors believe lasts anywhere between two minutes and four to six hours, the lack of blood and oxygen triggers a vicious cycle of increasing damage. Treatment is most effective if administered within this phase, which is why doctors urge people with stroke symptoms to seek immediate medical attention. In fact, stroke is now being called "brain attack," similar to "heart attack," to make the public more aware of the need for immediate recognition and prompt action. After the ischemic cascade, the brain goes through a reorganization phase, which lasts for about a week. After the reorganization, the brain enters a fairly stable phase, which may last anywhere from a week to three months. Preliminary results suggest that HBOT is not as useful during the reorganization phase as it is before or after this phase.

If the damaged area is not too large, or is not in a critical area, a person might recover spontaneously from a stroke. In some cases, what was originally thought to be a stroke turns out to have been a TIA. TIA recovery usually takes place within twenty-four hours, while stroke recovery generally occurs within the first couple of weeks after the attack. In unusual cases, spontaneous recovery may occur as long as three months after the attack. Most neurologists believe that little or no further recovery will occur after three months.

Many treatments are used to help people recover from strokes. Drugs are used to relieve various abnormal conditions, including spasm, high blood pressure, and brain swelling. Surgery is used to reduce spasticity, remove abnormal tissue, and lessen pressure within the skull. Some of the newer stroke-treatment methods include nutritional counseling, herbal medicine, acupuncture, and psychotherapy. Even spiritual healing has been attempted. Physical therapy is used to help the patient regain various functions and to encourage plasticity.

None of these methods are considered satisfactory. As a result, a certain pessimistic attitude pervades the medical profession when it comes to the treatment of stroke. However, the use of HBOT offers a more optimistic outlook for stroke patients and their loved ones.

HOW HBOT HELPS THE BRAIN RECOVER

As we have described, the most important factors in a stroke patient's recovery is the extent of the infarct and of the penumbra, the region that surrounds the infarct. The presence of viable brain tissue in the penumbra explains why the initial symptoms do not always predict how much function the patient can eventually recover.[2] Key attributes of HBOT are that it decreases swelling and reawakens the stunned neurons within the penumbra by providing them with oxygen.[3,4]

Activation of these neurons explains why patients can show improvement when HBOT is administered years after a stroke occurs—in some cases, up to thirteen years afterward.[5,6] Many stroke patients have stunned, but living, brain cells, which are especially common in cases where imaging studies show the presence of potentially recoverable brain tissue.[7]

The revival of nonfunctional neurons is HBOT's most notable effect in cases of stroke, but not its only effect. This therapy provides the stroke patient with a number of other benefits:

- *Relief of oxygen starvation.* Oxygen starvation, also known as hypoxia, occurs during ischemia, when the flow of blood is reduced. Since full blood circulation to an ischemic area cannot be restored immediately, the only way to get oxygen into the ischemic tissues is by increasing the rate at which oxygen diffuses into all of the body's fluids. HBOT increases the amount of oxygen carried to the tissues by forcing oxygen into the plasma (the liquid portion of the blood), the lymph, and the cerebrospinal fluid (the fluid that bathes the brain and spinal cord). If absolutely no blood can reach an area, as is the case in a complete arterial blockage, the oxygen-enriched cerebrospinal fluid will help to nurture the tissues.[8]

- *Improvement of microcirculation.* Microcirculation refers to the flow of blood through the capillaries, the tiny blood vessels that connect the arteries to the veins. The capillaries are where nutrients, including oxygen, leave the bloodstream and enter the tissues. Oxygenated tissues are also able to repair themselves by producing new capillaries.[9]

- *Relief of brain swelling.* Following a stroke, there is considerable swelling, also known as *edema,* of the brain. Drugs can reduce this swelling, but often have adverse effects on normal brain tissue. Swelling tends to recur after the patient stops taking the drugs. Moreover, although drugs can reduce edema, they cannot supply the brain with needed oxygen. HBOT safely reduces edema by causing the blood vessels to contract. Once the extra fluid around the brain cells is drained away, the cells can function more effectively. It also allows cell wastes to be more easily removed, which keeps the wastes from building up to toxic levels.[10]

- *Relief of spasticity.* A stroke patient's muscles often become spastic, or rigid. This spasticity becomes the greatest obstacle to proper physical therapy. HBOT has been proven to be an effective and nontoxic antispasticity measure. It is not clear how HBOT reduces spasticity, but it probably has something to do with the activation of neurons in the penumbra zone of the brain.

Treatment with HBOT has other benefits for the stroke patient. They include the reduction of free radicals, molecules that can cause tissue damage, and the stimulation of nerve impulses through the spinal cord where it meets the base of the brain.

Studies demonstrate HBOT's effectiveness in treating stroke. For instance, eight of nine animal studies showed positive results when HBOT was used.[11–18] In the one experimental failure, the authors admitted that an anesthetic used during surgery on that study's dogs could have nullified the effects of HBOT.[19]

Positive effects have also been reported in human patients. For example, in a study by Dr. K.H. Holbach and colleagues, 35 stroke patients had chronic artery blockages. These people were treated with HBOT an average of ten weeks after their strokes. HBOT was given to them at 1.5 atmospheres absolute (see "The Language of HBOT and of Research" on page 7) for forty minutes daily. Treatment continued for about two weeks. The patients were evaluated by clinical examination and by electroencephalogram (EEG), a test that measures brain waves.

Of the 35 subjects, 15 patients improved, both clinically and according to their EEGs, and underwent an operation called an extracranial/intracranial (EC/IC) arterial bypass. This operation, which provides the brain with extra blood flow, allowed these people to maintain their improvements. Another 15 patients did not improve after HBOT, and were not operated on. And 5 additional patients who did not improve with HBOT nevertheless underwent EC/IC bypass but still did not improve.[20]

HBOT also works well with physical therapy, in which exercise and other forms of movement are used to help a patient regain control of the limbs. Physical therapy reorganizes the neurons awakened by HBOT, allowing these neurons to regain their plasticity.

In another study, 122 patients with strokes caused by blood clots were treated with HBOT. Of the 122, 79 were treated from five months to ten years after their initial attacks—beyond the time that spontaneous recovery is believed to take place. Many of the patients had received various conventional physical therapies. They underwent HBOT at 1.5 to 2.0 atmospheres absolute, with duration and frequency of treatment adjusted as each patient improved. Of the 79 patients, 65 percent reported improvement in their quality of life. The HBOT patients spent much less time in the hospital—an average of 177 days compared with 287 days for conventionally treated patients. It is noteworthy that all of the HBOT patients were able to go home, while a number of the other patients had to enter rehabilitation centers. That represents a significant conservation of resources, in both emotional and financial terms, for the HBOT patients.[21]

In a study by noted hyperbaricist Dr. K.K. Jain, spasticity was reduced in a large percentage of patients who received HBOT. This improvement was made permanent when HBOT was used daily and combined with physical therapy.[22]

PICTURING THE POWER OF HBOT

Surviving the initial crisis of a stroke is only the beginning of a long recovery process. Before this process is undertaken, an accurate diagnosis must be made, one that shows the exact location and extent of the damage. That provides both the doctor and the patient with a baseline against which future progress can be measured.

Medical science has developed a number of imaging systems that give doctors the ability to see what is happening inside a patient's body without the risks of exploratory surgery (see "Peering Within the Body" on page 23). These systems have allowed doctors to learn more about how stroke affects the brain.

One of these systems, SPECT, is particularly useful in following the progress of patients treated with HBOT. Like other body-imaging systems, SPECT causes minimal discomfort for the patient. Before being scanned, the patient is injected with a minute amount of radioactive tracer. This tracer travels via the bloodstream to the brain, where it binds to active neurons. The patient is then positioned under a special camera that takes color pictures of the brain. These pictures show where the tracer has accumulated, which is where there are active neurons. SPECT can be used before and after an HBOT treatment to measure any improvement that may take place. In certain instances, such before-and-after scans show a large region of potentially recoverable brain tissue.[23]

Current literature indicates that the radioactive tracer used in SPECT poses minimal health risks to the patient. The total body radiation from a SPECT scan is less than that received from a chest x-ray or CAT scan. However, it is important for a patient to always discuss possible side effects from any procedure or medication with his or her own doctor, or the doctor supervising the procedure. One good reason not to undergo a SPECT scan is use of a monoamine oxidase (MAO) inhibitor within the previous fourteen days. Another reason is pregnancy.

Dr. Neubauer uses SPECT in his own practice to track patient progress. In one case, a 66-year-old man suffered a stroke that caused damage to his brain's frontal lobe and to the midbrain. As a result, he required the full-time care of his wife, at home. In all, only half of his brain was functioning (see Figure 2.1, Plate 1). After one hour of HBOT, it was obvious that recoverable tissue did exist (see Figure 2.2, Plate 1). Eventually, this patient went from almost total incapacitation to being able to speak, feed himself, maintain bowel control, and move with assistance. While not a complete recovery, the improvement in this patient's condition did represent a tremendous enhancement of his quality of life. It also lessened the physical, emotional, and financial burdens on the patient's family.

In another case, a 60-year-old woman had suffered a stroke thirteen years before receiving HBOT. A SPECT scan showed a large right-side infarct, which had left her with speech and drooling problems, as well as motion problems on her right side (Figure 2.3, Plate 2). The damaged area was surrounded with idlingneurons, cells that received enough oxygen to remain alive but not enough to function properly. She then received one session of HBOT, followed by another SPECT scan (Figure 2.4, Plate 3). Not only did the scan show improved brain function, but after a number of HBOT sessions, the muscles on the right side of the patient's body were less spastic, and she was able to walk more easily, although still with a cane. After a total of sixty HBOT treatments, the patient stopped drooling and was able to speak more clearly, and her ability to move continued to show improvement.[24] SPECT studies of brain-injured patients who were given oxygen at normal pressure showed that their penumbras did not become

Peering Within the Body

The ability of doctors to peer within the living body has improved dramatically since the development of x-rays in the late nineteenth century. *Computerized axial tomography* (CAT), also referred to as computerized tomography (CT), uses x-rays to produce a highly accurate picture of the structures within the body, and how those structures relate to one another. Tumors, blood clots, bone displacements, and fluid pools can be detected via CAT.

Another form of body imaging is *magnetic resonance imaging* (MRI), also known as nuclear magnetic resonance (NMR). MRI uses magnets and radio waves to produce images of organs and processes within the body. It was discovered that with MRI, changes in the brain could be seen much earlier than with CAT. Thus, the extent and severity of a stroke could be more accurately diagnosed. Another system, *magnetic resonance angiography* (MRA), is able to accurately map blood flow from the carotid artery in the neck all the way through the brain.

Yet another imaging system employs gamma rays to show what is happening within the body. *Positron emission tomography* (PET) is able to measure the brain's blood flow and function in just one scanning session. It also provides a sharp picture of the brain's anatomy, but is used primarily to determine function. Unfortunately, PET, an excellent system, is not often used because of its high cost.

Doctors now have a diagnostic system that is even more effective than previous systems in visualizing the extent and nature of stroke damage. This system is known as *single photon emission computerized tomography* (SPECT). In a similar manner to the PET scan, SPECT can depict the actual functioning of the living brain.

nearly as activated as those of patients who received oxygen at appropriate hyperbaric pressures.[25]

Timely treatment of stroke is very important, since the chances of recovery are greatest if treatment is administered within the acute phase, the first phase after a stroke occurs (see page 16). HBOT should begin at 1.5 atmospheres absolute (see "The Language of HBOT and of Research" on page 7), increasing to 1.75 atmospheres absolute if necessary. Pressures above 1.75 are rarely used. Therapy should be administered for one hour every six hours around the clock until the stroke is stabilized, which generally requires about thirty treatments in total.

HBOT can be used with tissue plasminogen activator (TPA), a drug that breaks up blood clots. While TPA is a useful adjunct in the treatment of acute stroke, it does have its drawbacks. First, it must be used within three hours after a stroke begins. Since many strokes occur at night, often at least eight hours pass before a stroke is diagnosed. Second, TPA can cause either early or delayed bleeding, and should therefore never be used for strokes caused by bleeding. Third, it takes three months after TPA is administered to learn whether or not it has worked. Pharmaceutical companies are working on drugs that can be used at a later stage in a stroke, and that produce fewer side effects.

HBOT can also be used with a newly developed operation that pumps oxygen-rich blood from a large artery in the patient's groin through a tube into the veins of the neck. This allows doctors to bypass the clogged artery. HBOT is also effective when used with another operation called an omentum transposition (see page 35).

HBOT can also be used with various types of rehabilitative measures, including physical, speech, and occupational therapies; computerized brain jogging; and biofeedback.

Practicing neurologists are slowly coming to agree with the idea of identifying stroke-affected brain tissue that might be recoverable. It is accepted medical practice that every measure should be taken to help awaken the dormant neurons within the damaged tissue and thus restore each patient to as much of that individual's prestroke capacity as possible. The use of HBOT as part of a comprehensive treatment plan is the simplest and most effective way of doing just that. In the next chapter, we'll learn how HBOT can be used to help treat other types of brain injuries.

CHAPTER 3

Using HBOT to Treat Central Nervous System and Sensory Problems

In Brazil, 17-year-old Maria V. has been in a wheelchair since coming out of coma fourteen years ago following a near-drowning. She cannot stand without being propped up, and suffers from mental retardation. Maria undergoes fifty-two HBOT sessions, after which her speech, comprehension, coordination, and hand movement are much improved. After more than 200 treatments, she can walk up the stairs with support, and speaks both Spanish and English.

Every year, more than 150,000 Americans suffer severe head injuries. Like stroke, head injuries deprive certain areas of the brain of oxygen. Again, as in the case of stroke, the damage resembles an atomic bomb blast, with a central core of what is probably irreparable damage surrounded by a penumbra of lesser damage. It is both the size and location of the initial damage, as well as the reversibility of the damage within the penumbra, that dictates the patient's prognosis. In some cases, this damage can be reversed by HBOT.

But head injury isn't the only cause of brain damage. Every year, thousands of Americans suffer brain damage as the result of near-hanging, near-drowning, near-choking, cardiac arrest, cyanide and carbon monoxide poisonings, and lightning strikes. This type of brain damage is known as anoxic ischemic encephalopathy. In this chapter, we'll look at how HBOT can help get oxygen to the injured brain. (Poisoning is treated more thoroughly in Chapter 10.)

Every year, more than 7,200 Americans suffer paralyzing spinal cord injuries. HBOT can also aid some of these people, since hyperbaric oxygen can help to revive nerve cells in the spinal cord in the same way it can help stimulate nerve cells in the brain. (The brain and spinal cord together make up the central nervous system.)

In addition, HBOT can assist in the alleviation of migraine headaches, and in the treatment of various eye and ear problems. (See Appendix A for information on contacting hyperbaric oxygen facilities.)

HBOT AND THE INJURED BRAIN

Brain damage often occurs after a head injury because the brain starts to swell, pressing delicate tissue against the unyielding skull. One researcher found that 80 percent of patients with serious head injuries had brain swelling. This swelling leads to a vicious cycle: the swelling cuts off the brain's blood supply, which leads to the accumulation of toxic levels of normal cell wastes. These wastes, in turn, further aggravate the swelling. Such damage can lead to *coma*, a state of deep unconsciousness in which the patient does not respond to pain or sound, and cannot be awakened. But even under such circumstances, certain brain cells survive in a dormant state within the zone between the damaged and the healthy parts of the brain, a zone called the penumbra. (See Chapter 2 for a complete discussion of this topic, and of other factors important to brain-injury recovery.)

HBOT can, at times, break this cycle by constricting the brain's blood vessels, yet delivering more oxygen. This seems like a contradiction, but HBOT can increase oxygen levels because the increased pressure forces oxygen into the blood plasma, the liquid part of the blood that normally does not carry oxygen, and into the cerebrospinal fluid that surrounds the brain. The plasma and cerebrospinal fluid can then reach areas that the red blood cells, which normally carry oxygen, cannot penetrate. With HBOT, oxygen in the capillaries is pushed further into the adjacent tissues than when oxygen is administered at standard pressure. HBOT can also stabilize and repair what is called the *blood-brain barrier*, a protective layer of cells that keeps many toxins or noxious materials from reaching the brain. This barrier is often greatly disturbed when a head injury occurs.[1]

As a result of the extra oxygen that HBOT provides, the dormant brain cells in the penumbra are awakened and begin to function again. Giving a patient pure oxygen at normal pressure simply cannot put enough oxygen into either the bloodstream or the cerebrospinal fluid to overcome the oxygen deficit. But HBOT can improve this oxygen deficiency.[2] Often, this increased oxygenation helps to restore the patient to a conscious state.[3] In certain cases, it also allows the patient to recover from brain-damage aftereffects such as paralysis and speech loss.

Unfortunately, standard emergency care for head injury generally does not include HBOT. Sometimes, the patient's condition deteriorates while the doctors are trying to find out what's wrong. In many cases, pressure within the skull is not monitored for signs of swelling. Steroids are occasionally given in an effort to reduce brain swelling. However, side effects of these drugs include an increase in the chance of infection and the formation of stomach ulcers. Most trauma centers hyperventilate the patient, making the person breathe rapidly and shallowly through the use of a ventilator. Hyperventilation is supposed to reduce pressure within the head. However, most brain specialists consider this practice dangerous because it reduces blood flow to the brain. As a result of these inadequate procedures, and depending on the degree of trauma, patients are often left with permanent brain damage because the underlying problem is not properly understood and treated.[4]

The use of HBOT in emergency situations can reduce

the chances of permanent damage. A 1987 study by Dr. D. Mathieu and colleagues analyzed the cases of 136 patients who received HBOT after trying to hang themselves. A fairly high pressure of 2.5 atmospheres absolute was used (see "The Language of HBOT and of Research" on page 7) in a monoplace chamber. Each session lasted ninety minutes, and the sessions were repeated at six-hour intervals until each responding individual regained consciousness. All patients received pure oxygen at normal pressure between HBOT sessions.

Of the 136 patients, 77.5 percent recovered without lasting aftereffects. Five percent recovered, but suffered neurological problems, while 17.5 percent died. The important factor was the time lapse between when the patient was found and when HBOT was started. If HBOT was given before the third hour after hanging, 85 percent of the patients recovered without neurological aftereffects. If HBOT was delayed for more than three hours, only 56 percent of the patients recovered without any aftereffects.[5]

Prompt use of HBOT is important because the more time a patient spends in a coma, the poorer his or her chances are of making a good recovery. In a 1981 study of 24 patients who survived at least one month in a coma, only 5 were alive at the end of a year. Three patients remained in permanent comas, while 2 came out of their comas with overwhelming disabilities.[6] Reports of other researchers generally indicate a similarly poor outlook for patients who remain in a coma after one month.[7]

However, there is evidence that HBOT can aid comatose patients, even patients who have been in prolonged comas. Doctors can use SPECT scanning to identify treatable brain tissue. Many times, brain tissue contains brain cells that have been stunned but not killed outright, and HBOT can revive some of these cells (see Chapter 2 for a fuller explanation).

Evidence of HBOT's effectiveness in treating brain damage was first published in a 1964 report from the Netherlands by Dr. V.A. Fasano and colleagues.[8] In 1985, Dr.

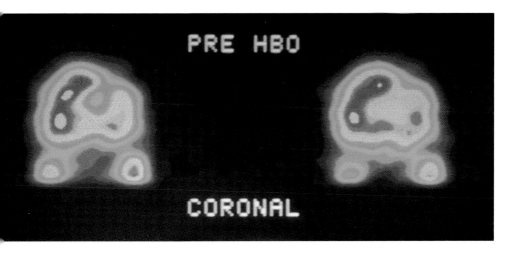

Figure 2.1.
This SPECT scan of a male 66-year-old stroke patient shows damage in the frontal lobe and the midbrain. This produced speech problems, some difficulty in swallowing, and weakness on the left side of the body.

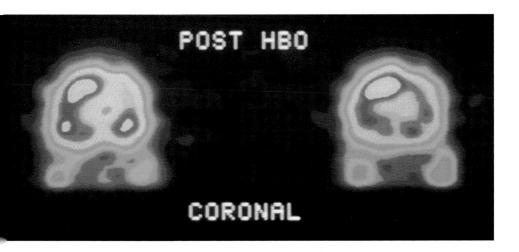

Figure 2.2.
This scan, taken after one HBOT session, shows areas of recoverable brain tissue. After a series of HBOT treatments, the patient became more mobile, had more energy, was able to maintain bowel control, and was able to feed himself and to speak.

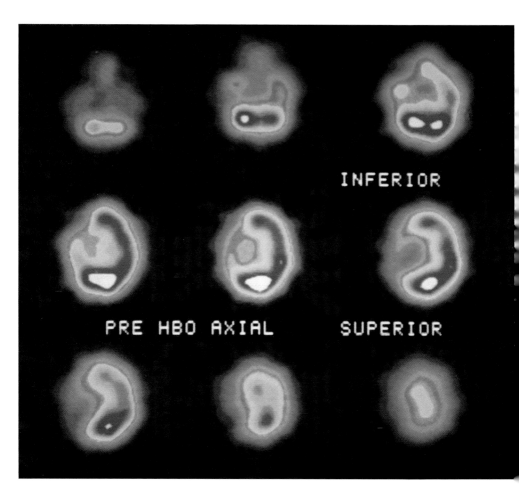

Figure 2.3.

This SPECT scan of a female 60-year-old stroke patient was taken thirteen years after the stroke occurred. It shows a large infarct on the right side of the brain, which produced drooling, and problems with speech and motion.

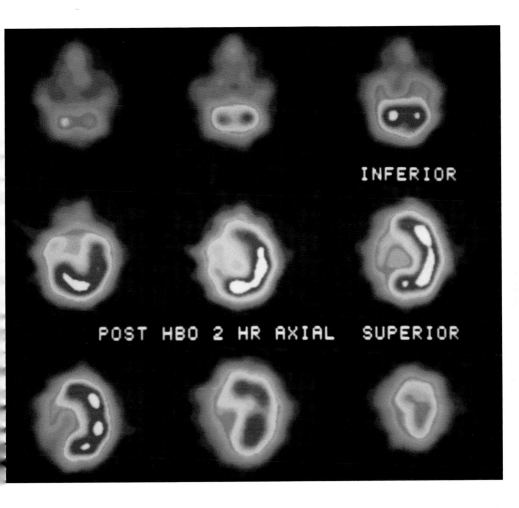

Figure 2.4.

This scan, taken after one HBOT session, shows improved brain function. After additional sessions, the patient stopped drooling and spoke more clearly, and was able to move more easily.

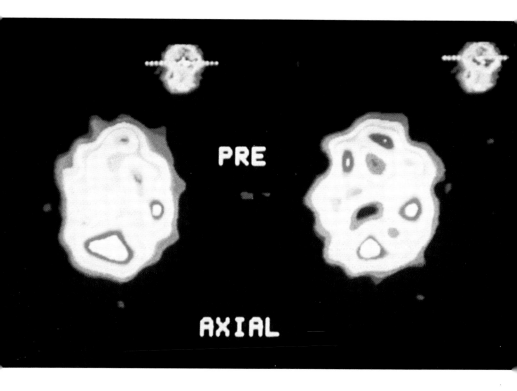

Figure 3.1.

This SPECT scan of a male 15-year-old head-injury patient shows damaged areas throughout the brain, including fluid accumulation and bruising. This damage produced problems with speech, motion, and memory.

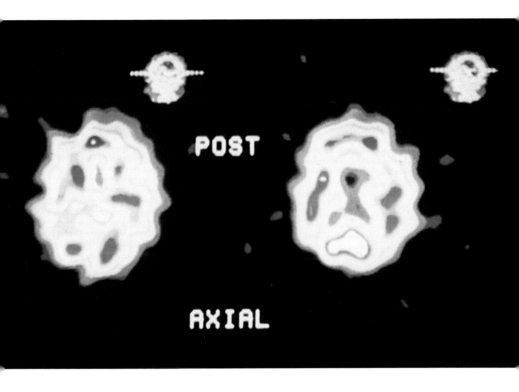

Figure 3.2.

This scan, taken after one HBOT session, shows great improvement in appearance. After additional sessions, the patient regained nearly normal function.

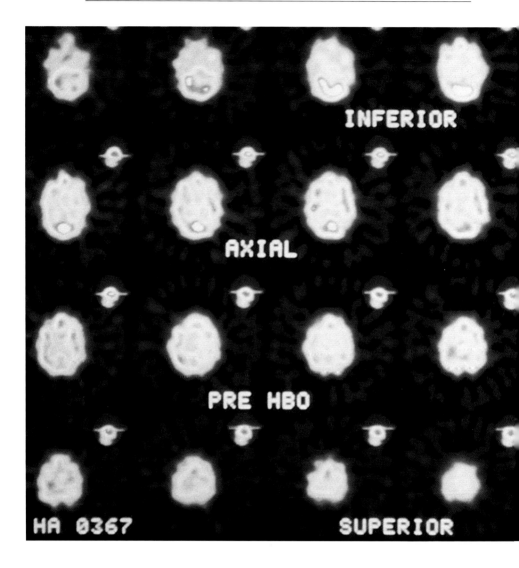

Figure 3.3.

This SPECT scan is of a male 19-year-old patient who had suffered by carbon monoxide poisoning. It shows extensive brain damage.

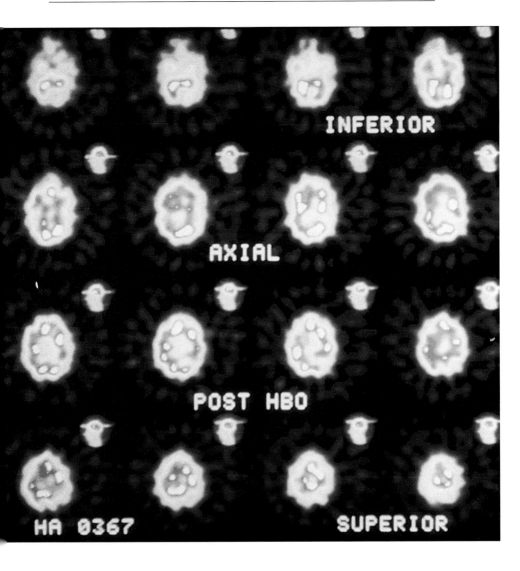

Figure 3.4.

This scan, taken after one HBOT session, shows great improvement in appearance. After additional sessions, the patient was able to act on his preaccident plans by going to college.

Neubauer published a case study on 20 comatose patients. The patients ranged in age from three years to sixty-seven years, and their comas ranged in duration from three to twenty-seven months. These patients were given between 80 and 120 sessions of HBOT at pressures that varied from 1.5 to 1.75 atmospheres absolute. Fifty percent of these patients improved substantially, and of these, 35 percent became self-sufficient. Improvement sometimes came slowly, in some cases not appearing until eighty treatments or more had been given. Only one patient showed postcoma psychosis, a mental illness that sometimes occurs after a person comes out of a coma. Postcoma psychosis is known to occur at a much higher rate for coma patients who are not treated with HBOT.[9,10]

In another study, 17 comatose children were given HBOT. The published report strongly suggests that hyperbaric oxygen helped these patients.[11]

Many animal studies have been done to evaluate the effects of HBOT on brain damage. However, some of these studies have been badly flawed. For example, a 1986 study involved three groups of dogs with cardiac arrest. One group, the control group, received no treatment. Another group received blood dilution, which thins the blood. The third group received the blood dilution plus one session of HBOT at 2.0 atmospheres absolute. No significant differences were noted among the three groups of dogs.[12] This result is not surprising, since no one could expect a single HBOT session to exert much of a beneficial effect.

In Chapter 2, we saw how a powerful body-imaging system called SPECT has allowed doctors to document the increase in brain function brought about by HBOT. Two cases serve as dramatic examples. One case involves a 15-year-old Texas boy who suffered a serious head injury in a motor vehicle accident. He underwent surgery for removal of a blood clot on the brain and afterward remained semicomatose for several months. He was then transferred to a rehabilitation center. There, he made progress to a point, but could not talk or walk, and continued to suffer from poor memory and decreased attention span.

The patient's parents took him to a hyperbaric facility. Tests, including SPECT, showed damage throughout the brain, including excessive fluid accumulation and bruising (see Figure 3.1, Plate 4).

After just one HBOT session, the function of the boy's brain was greatly improved (see Figure 3.2, Plate 5). The patient then received twenty HBOT sessions at 1.5 atmospheres absolute. Again, the improvement was substantial. There were daily increases in the boy's attention span, alertness, and ability to use language. His leg muscles became much less spastic, which improved the response to physical therapy. When he returned to the rehabilitation facility in Texas, he was able to name by title, for the first time since his admission, all of the professionals attending him. He took further treatments at a nearby hyperbaric facility and was released. Eventually, the boy was able to attend his high school graduation dance.

Another example is Heraldo P., who was overcome by natural gas fumes from his home's water heater while taking a shower. He lapsed into a coma. When he awoke twenty days later, the 19-year-old prelaw student had the thinking capacity of a 12-year-old and severe problems with muscle movement. For two years afterward, Heraldo showed no physical or mental improvement.

At that point, Heraldo's parents took him from their home in Brazil to Dr. Neubauer's facility in Florida. Heraldo underwent a SPECT study before treatment, and it showed extensive brain damage (Figure 3.3, Plate 6). The appearance of his brain showed considerable improvement after one HBOT treatment (Figure 3.4, Plate 7). Because of this change for the better, Heraldo received nineteen treatments, one hour each at 1.5 atmospheres absolute, and continued to make rapid improvement. Treatments would have continued, but Heraldo's visa expired, and he and his parents returned to Brazil.

Heraldo's mental capacity continued to improve at home

even without any additional HBOT treatments. Six months later, the family called Dr. Neubauer to say that because of the young man's progress, he had reentered the university.

HBOT shows striking results when a pressure of 1.5 atmospheres absolute is used in one-hour sessions. The total dose of HBOT depends on the needs of each patient. Frequency can vary from one to three times a day, and the total number of sessions can vary widely. However, increasing pressure to 2.0 atmospheres absolute may be potentially harmful, so the hyperbaricist has to be careful in administering HBOT.[13,14] It is important to see HBOT as part of a long-term rehabilitation plan. Such a plan should include other therapies, such as physical therapy, occupational therapy, speech therapy, and computerized brain jogging (computer software that allows the patient to exercise various mental functions). HBOT is also effective when used with an operation called an omentum transposition (see page 35).

HBOT AND SPINAL CORD PROBLEMS

The spinal cord is made up of similar types of nerve tissue to that found in the brain. Therefore, when it is bruised, it tends to undergo the same type of damage to which the brain is subject. That is, swelling causes a cutoff of the blood supply, which in turn causes the cells to die from lack of oxygen and from being poisoned by their own waste. This process can lead to permanent disability below the affected section of cord. An injury that occurs high on the spine, such as in the neck, may also leave the patient with bladder and bowel control problems, in addition to paralysis of the extremities.

Sometimes, a severe spinal cord bruise produces a *physiological transection,* in which the swelling, lack of oxygen, and production of toxins causes the cord to transect itself. A transected cord is as bad as a severed cord, in that no nerve impulses can pass through the transection.

Within the damaged areas, many nerve cells remain alive. However, they are often stunned into inactivity (see Chapter 2 for a fuller discussion). HBOT can reduce swelling and overcome a lack of oxygen in the nerve tissues of the spinal cord. This increased oxygenation allows the stunned nerve cells to become active once more.

If the injury is severe enough to actually sever the cord, there is little that can be done to restore function. If the cord has not been severed, it is possible that HBOT can reduce the swelling to the point that permanent paralysis does not develop. However, HBOT must be used within one to six hours after the injury for it to have any chance of completely reversing the damage.

Other disorders can affect the spinal cord. Of these disorders, the following conditions respond well to HBOT:

- Air embolism, in which an air bubble blocks circulation (see Chapter 1 for more information on air embolism)

- Stroke that affects the spine (see Chapter 2 for more information on stroke)

- Decompression sickness involving the spinal cord (see Chapter 1 for more information on decompression sickness)

A number of studies have shown HBOT's effectiveness in cases where spinal damage is associated with injuries.[15-20] In these studies, HBOT showed an ability to improve blood flow to the spinal cord, to reduce swelling, and to correct disturbances in various bodily chemicals. In an animal study at Texas A&M University, rats with severed spinal cords showed some return of nerve function after between forty-seven and fifty-four HBOT treatments. Further improvement was seen among rats that were treated with both HBOT and dimethyl sulfoxide (DMSO).[21] (Doctors are not optimistic that this would happen in humans.) And in a 1985 Soviet study, 43 patients with reduced spinal blood flow showed improvement after HBOT was administered. A control group of similar patients was given drugs that dilated their blood vessels, but did not receive HBOT. These latter patients did not show any improvement.[22]

There are some situations in which the spinal cord has obviously been bruised, such as in the case of a patient who has struck his or her head on the bottom of a swimming pool while diving. In these cases, the patient should be placed in the hyperbaric chamber immediately, before any tests or imaging studies are done. The prompt use of HBOT can help prevent permanent paralysis. The ideal treatment for spinal cord injury would be one hour of HBOT at 1.5 atmospheres absolute every six hours until the injury is stabilized, for a total of between 20 and 100 treatments (see "The Language of HBOT and of Research" on page 7). Tests that measure the flow of nerve impulses between the brain and the extremities can be helpful in guiding such treatment. A recently developed procedure called an *omentum transposition* gives doctors a new way to treat spinal cord injuries. In the abdominal cavity, there is a membrane, called the omentum, which hangs from the stomach. It contains a rich supply of neurotransmitters, the chemicals that carry nerve impulses between nerve cells, and of growth factors for both blood vessels and nerves. In an omentum transposition, surgeons tailor this membrane so that it is quite long, but still attached. It can then be brought under the skin to the spinal cord and laid directly on the affected area. Blood vessels will grow from the omentum into the spinal cord, bringing in an additional blood flow, as well as a rich supply of neurotransmitters and growth factors. This procedure can also be done with strokes and brain injuries.

HBOT works well with omentum transposition. In fact, HBOT provides a good screening technique, since people who improve after receiving HBOT are likely to improve after this surgical procedure.

HBOT also works well with physical therapy, since physical therapy gives a pattern, or sense of direction, to the stunned neurons newly awakened by HBOT. It may also reduce spasticity, or muscle rigidity, which is a major hurdle to rehabilitation,[23] and can aid quadriplegics and paraplegics by relieving bedsores (see Chapter 9).

HBOT AND MIGRAINE HEADACHES

Many severe, intractable, recurrent headaches are labeled migraine headaches. In fact, "migraine headache" has become a household term. However, the classic migraine, which can last for hours, is a specific type of headache that may incapacitate the person who suffers from it. Attacks often begin with sensory disturbances, such as flashing lights or strange odors, along with nausea and vomiting. The actual headache itself brings severe pain on one side of the head, generally beginning in or around one eye, and sensitivity to light. Afterwards, the affected person may have dull neck and head pains, and may be quite sleepy.

Migraines are vascular headaches, or headaches caused by changes in blood flow to and within the brain. Although migraines represent only 8 percent of all headaches, these and other vascular headaches tend to make people quite ill and often require medical attention.[24] A migraine headache begins with constriction of blood vessels in the brain. During the first phase of a migraine, blood flow may be reduced by an average of 36 percent.[25] The specific symptoms that are experienced as a result of this reduced blood flow—such as visions of flashing lights—depend on which area of the brain is affected.[26]

Reduced blood flow results in a lack of oxygen in the tissues, along with changes in the brain's chemistry. This, in turn, causes the release of substances that greatly dilate the blood vessels. Local tissue injury and swelling occur as a result. It is at this time that migraine pain strikes the patient.[27]

Because administered oxygen constricts the blood vessels while oxygenating the tissues, HBOT can reduce swelling by as much as 50 percent. This aborts the symptoms. In a study by Dr. William Fife and Dr. Caroline Fife, HBOT was given to 26 patients who had migraine headache pain. Pressures between 1.3 and 2.4 atmospheres absolute were used (see "The Language of HBOT and of Research" on page 7) in a multiplace chamber. All but one patient obtained complete relief of migraine symptoms within minutes of exposure, including two patients who had temporary paralysis on one side of the face before HBOT treatment.[28]

Relief of symptoms occurs as quickly as five minutes after the migraine patient starts to breathe pure oxygen at between 1.3 and 1.75 atmospheres absolute. Occasionally, a pressure of 2 atmospheres absolute may be needed.[29–31] Increased amounts of oxygen in the blood raise oxygen levels in the brain tissues, even when contracted blood vessels reduce blood flow. Many migraine patients who receive HBOT find that the interval between attacks is significantly increased.

HBOT AND SENSORY PROBLEMS

Reductions in blood flow and loss of nerve function can cause various problems with hearing and/or vision. HBOT has been used successfully to treat these kinds of problems.

How HBOT Eases Ear Problems

The inner ear contains a rich supply of blood vessels and nerves, all of which are very sensitive to trauma, infection, illness, toxins, and reductions in blood flow. Any one of these factors, or any combination of them, can cause a loss of hearing and sometimes balance. HBOT has been used to treat various ear problems, including tinnitus, sudden deafness, acoustic trauma, and Ménière's disease.

Tinnitus—a tinkling, buzzing, hissing, or ringing sound heard in one or both ears—is the most common symptom associated with inner-ear damage.[32] Doctors are not entirely sure what causes tinnitus. It is thought to be related to circulation problems involving the inner ear, a cone-shaped organ responsible for both hearing and balance. Blood vessels leading to the inner ear may become partially blocked, which reduces blood flow to the sensitive nerves related to hearing. However, tinnitus can occur in nearly all disorders of the ear, including infections, obstructions, and tumors. It may also occur as the result of cardiovascular disease, poisoning, or head injury.[33] Tinnitus is sometimes treated by implanting an electrode in the patient's head that emits a sound at a deeper pitch than the patient usually hears. That seems to block out the tinnitus in some cases.

Every year, about 1 in 5,000 persons will suffer from sudden hearing loss, or hearing loss that develops in one ear over a period of several hours. As in the case of tinnitus, its cause is not always known. The oldest explanation for this disorder is that it is due to decreased blood flow. However, it may be related to viral infections, diabetes, high cholesterol levels, poisoning, diving injuries, noise, or rupture of membranes in the ear.

Acoustic traum is defined as sudden hearing impairment caused by sharp sounds, such as a gun going off near an unprotected ear. Sounds of moderate intensity, such as those encountered in everyday life, usually do not cause acoustic trauma.

Ménière's disease is recognized as a separate clinical entity. The standard symptoms are roaring tinnitus, espisodes of dizziness, and fluctuating hearing loss. A typical attack is followed by nausea and vomiting.

The conventional medical treatment for these ear problems employs drugs that dilate the blood vessels in an effort to improve blood circulation. Steroids and vitamins have also been administered. However, such treatments rarely work and may sometimes be harmful.[34,35]

One treatment that has shown itself to be useful is HBOT. There are two reasons. One is that HBOT increases the oxygen concentration in the inner ear.[36] The other is that hyperbaric oxgyen improves the flexibility of the red blood cells, thereby improving the microcirculation in the affected area.[37]

One of the first studies on HBOT and ear disorders was reported in 1969, in which 33 patients with reduced inner-ear blood flow improved after receiving HBOT.[38] Other studies show similar results: 8 patients with tinnitus or partial deafness had their hearing improved by HBOT;[39] and 12 patients who were treated with HBOT experienced marked hearing improvement.[40] In yet another study, 107 patients had transient ischemia, or intermittent blood-flow blockages in the artery leading to the ear. They received HBOT at 1.5 to 2.0 atmospheres absolute (see "The Language of HBOT and of Research" on page 7) in sessions of thirty-five or forty minutes daily for eight to ten days, and achieved good results.[41] Further studies have shown HBOT to be of some benefit in cases of Ménière's disease.[42] It should be noted that the medical literature on the use of HBOT for ear diseases is not extensive.

Best results are achieved if HBOT is started as early as possible after the onset of deafness. The spontaneous recovery rate, which is as high as 90 percent, makes both the selection of patients for treatment and the evaluation of results particularly difficult.[43] It is important to test the patient for any underlying causes, such as infections, tumors, or injuries, where other therapies may have significant importance.

In cases of acoustic trauma, the patient should receive HBOT within the first three days of the espisode. A pressure of 2.5 atmospheres absolute should be used in ten one-hour sessions, a session per day for ten days. In cases of tinnitus or deafness from other causes, there are several different treatment plans.

How HBOT Eases Macular Degeneration

There is some evidence that HBOT can reverse an eye disease called age-related macular degeneration (AMD), the leading cause of severe visual loss in people over the age of fifty. Macular degeneration is a wasting of either the optic nerve or the macula, a spot on the retina, which is the membrane in the back of the eye that receives images from the outside. The macula is the spot where vision is most acute. AMD appears as a painless loss of acuity in the center of the visual field, with the first symptom being visual distortion in one eye. There is frequently bleeding or excessive pigmentation in the macular region as the disease progresses. Eventually, the patient goes blind.

In a study by Dr. L. Bojic and colleagues, 4 patients who had nearly total loss of eyesight from macular degeneration received HBOT. Three of the patients experienced a doubling of visual acuity, while the fourth experienced almost a fourfold increase in acuity. The doctors who treated the patients thought that the hyperbaric oxygen helped increase the amount of oxygen in the retinal tissue, which allowed the retina to renew itself without causing a buildup of waste material. They thought this waste material interfered with cell function and led to macular degeneration.[44]

The use of HBOT in the treatment of AMD requires more research. However, a treatment plan can be suggested based on preliminary results: thirty ninety-minute sessions in thirty days at 2.0 atmospheres absolute, using a multiplace chamber. HBOT can be used along with other forms of treatment, such as laser therapy.

HBOT can drastically affect treatment of injuries to the brain, spinal cord, and sensory organs. In the next chapter, we'll see how HBOT can have an equally dramatic effect on multiple sclerosis.

CHAPTER 4

Using HBOT to Treat Multiple Sclerosis

In Florida, 38-year-old Teresa S. has been affected by multiple sclerosis for twenty-two years. Teresa has received HBOT on nearly a bimonthly basis since 1982, and has progressed steadily in her ongoing remission. "I was in a walker and then I walked with two canes, then one, and now I've thrown away both of them. HBO[T] just worked for me," she says. "I had refused to believe it until it actually worked. I've experienced so many false hopes before."

In Chapters 2 and 3, we saw how HBOT can help some patients to recover from disorders of the brain and spinal cord. In this chapter, we'll see how HBOT can help improve the lives of some patients who have multiple sclerosis (MS), another neurological disorder. There are approximately half a million MS patients in the United States, with about 10,000 Americans newly diagnosed each year. But there may be more people with MS than these figures indicate, because it is a diagnosis reached only after many other conditions are considered. While MS is generally not fatal, it can cause severe disability, including problems with motion, speech, and vision, and problems with bowel and bladder control.

HBOT has been documented as an important weapon in the fight against MS. In this chapter, we'll first describe and define what MS is, and take a look at differing theories about its cause. We'll then see how MS patients and their doctors can use HBOT to treat this crippling disease.

WHAT IS MULTIPLE SCLEROSIS?

In MS, the nerve fibers in the brain and spinal cord gradually lose their protective covering, which is made of a fatty substance called *myelin*. Nerve impulses are basically electrical impulses, so myelin covers and insulates a nerve in the same way insulation covers an electrical wire. A nerve that is covered with myelin conducts impulses more rapidly than a nerve that isn't covered. Therefore, when a nerve loses its myelin, signals do not travel through it properly. Just like a wire that loses its insulation, a nerve affected by MS develops a short circuit.

As a result of MS, hardened, scarred patches called *plaques* may develop throughout the brain and spinal cord, although affected areas do not always form plaques. Symptoms vary from patient to patient, and from time to time in the same patient, depending on where these plaques occur and how extensive they are.[1] Yet, even before these scars develop, MS can cause swelling and a lack of oxygen in the tissues which, in turn, can produce many different symptoms. Sometimes, these disturbed areas may heal spontaneously without plaque formation. Because of such spontaneous remissions, a firm evaluation of the patient's condition cannot be made for at least two years.

Women tend to suffer from MS more often than men. People who live in cold climates seem to develop it more frequently, in Minnesota and Michigan in particular. Although the disease tends to occur more commonly among relatives of people who already have it, there is no clear hereditary pattern.

MS begins slowly, usually in young adulthood, and continues throughout life. The first symptoms are numbness or abnormal sensations in the arms and legs or on one side of the face. Other early signs are sight disturbances such as double vision and partial blindness, muscle weakness, and dizziness. Later in the course of the disease there may be blurred vision, loss of muscle control, partial paralysis, abnormal reflexes, slurred speech, and urinary difficulties.

MS may cause a number of secondary problems, such as inflammation of the membranes covering the brain and spinal cord, problems with nerves beyond the brain and spinal cord, changes in the retina, loss of nerve cells, blood spots in the skin, and blood vessel changes.[2-7]

MS occurs in one of two patterns. The first pattern, the *relapsing/remitting* type, affects most people with MS. During a relapse, the disease is active and the nerves are damaged. As a result, new symptoms may appear or existing ones may worsen. The relapse may last for only a few days, or it may continue for several months. In a remission, the disease is quiet, although it may continue to progress without symptoms. Also, during remission, symptoms could be present because of damage previously done to the nerves. They may improve, but do not entirely disappear. After each relapse, the patient loses a little more ground.[8]

The second pattern is the *chronic and progressive* pattern, experienced by about 18 percent of all MS patients. In this pattern, there is a gradual worsening of symptoms over many years, without relapses or remissions. Symptoms may fluctuate, but, in general, advance steadily with a continually worsening prognosis.

People with MS sometimes experience impairments in their thinking ability. They are at times subject to mood swings and other emotional difficulties. They may feel angry, frightened, worried, or beyond hope. Denial—a state in which the patient tries to ignore the disease—is common. The patient may think, with some justification, that revealing his or her degree of anger or fear might be more than family or close friends can accept. On the other hand, family members frequently look desperately for advice on how to best assist the patient. In fact, because of the anxiety of both patients and their families, few other diseases have been the subject of such a variety of treatments.

THE CAUSES OF MS

No one is yet sure of what causes MS. However, a number of theories have been developed over the years, including a more recent theory developed by Dr. Neubauer and his colleague, Dr. Sheldon Gottlieb. We will first examine some of the other theories, after which we will discuss the Gottlieb-Neubauer theory.

Conventional Theories About the Cause of MS

A variety of treatments have been developed in an effort to reverse, or at least relieve, the symptoms of MS. These come out of two theories about what causes MS—viral infection and autoimmune dysfunction. Numerous investigators have done studies in which neither theory was found to be valid.[9-11] We also believe these theories are mistaken, and that they have delayed the search for proper MS therapy. To understand why this is so, it is important to examine these theories.

The viral theory states that the body reacts to an inflammation caused by a virus. However, before any microorganism can be said to cause a disease, the following scientific conditions must exist:

1. The microorganism must be present in all cases of the disease.
2. The microorganism must be isolated and grown in a pure culture outside of the body.
3. The cultured microorganism must produce the same disease in test animals.
4. The microorganism must be recovered, or reisolated, from the test animals and grown in pure culture.

All efforts to isolate a virus from the bodies of MS patients, according to the conditions stated above, have been unsuccessful.[12,13] Biopsies of active lesions have failed to yield any viable viruses. Not a single virus has been shown to meet these conditions. Therefore, there is no direct evidence that a virus starts the disease process associated with MS, nor is there evidence that a virus is a persistent part of the unfolding course of the disease. Still, the continued support for this theory has hindered the growth and exploration of competing theories.

The autoimmune dysfunction theory states that MS develops when the body, in essence, becomes allergic to itself. The immune system attacks the nerves, which results in loss of the myelin covering. However, this theory assumes that such damage is limited to the brain and spinal cord only, and not to nerves elsewhere. Such an assumption is disproven by the fact that nerves elsewhere in the body can be affected.[14]

There are other theories about why multiple sclerosis strikes. One holds that fat particles may become lodged within the blood vessels of the brain, creating a blockage in the circulation. This lack of circulation causes swelling, which in turn causes lesions to form.[15] Others believe an environmental factor is at work.[16] This approach includes the idea that MS is caused by a toxin, such as too much zinc resulting from occupational exposure.[17] Mercury is another circulating toxin suspected of inducing MS. Thus, MS patients have been replacing their mercury amalgam dental fillings with fillings made of other materials, such as porcelain, composite, or gold, to halt the progression of symptoms. Some people do have adverse responses to certain dental materials, including silver, tin, zinc, mercury, and copper. But the idea that such fillings can cause or aggravate MS is still open to question.

Why have these theories been vigorously pursued, despite a lack of evidence to support them? We believe this has happened because, after so much research time and money have been invested in them, people are reluctant to seriously examine other options.

Another Theory About the Cause of MS

There is another theory about what causes MS, a theory that explains why HBOT is proving to be such a successful treatment. This theory was developed by Dr. Neubauer, in conjunction with Dr. Sheldon Gottlieb of the University of South Alabama, through a combination of clinical observation and a detailed reading of the medical literature. It explains the inefficiency of available MS treatment methods. Together, the doctors published an extensive critical review of the world's medical and scientific literature in which they compared and contrasted the various ideas concerning the causes of MS. They also weighed the pluses and minuses of HBOT, and concluded that HBOT was the safest and most effective treatment available for MS.

What would lead them to this conclusion? Dr. Neubauer and Dr. Gottlieb believe that MS is a wound in the central nervous system (the brain and spinal cord taken together). They think this wound arises when blood pressure becomes elevated within the brain and spinal cord, and remains elevated for a prolonged period of time. This period of high blood pressure damages blood vessels that are genetically susceptible to such impairment. The damage, in turn, produces changes within the nerve tissue that results in a lack of oxygen, or hypoxia, similar to that seen in stroke and other forms of brain damage (see Chapters 2 and 3). In the case of MS, though, the hypoxia leads to the destruction of the nerve fibers' myelin sheaths, and to secondary damage associated with the immune system.[18]

This means that MS can be seen in the same light as stroke and other forms of brain and spinal cord damage— as being caused by a lack of oxygen within the body's tissues. Therefore, if HBOT can help put enough oxygen into the tissues to overcome the effects of stroke, it should be able to do the same thing for MS.

Dr. Neubauer and Dr. Gottlieb have found support among other health care professionals. Letters from doctors published in *The Lancet*, a well-respected British medical journal, indicate that there is evidence that MS is a disease of the blood vessels within the central nervous system. These writers tend to agree with the Gottlieb-Neubauer theory.[19-21]

USING HBOT TO TREAT MS

Existing drug therapies for MS can cause significant side effects that may be worse than the discomforts they are designed to relieve. A number of different drugs are used in MS therapy, including interferons and various steroids. These drugs not only cause a wide variety of side effects, but can be very expensive as well. Certain drug therapies can cost more than $25,000 a year.

HBOT is the only treatment that offers the MS patient relief of symptoms with no serious side effects. Unlike most of the other therapies, it is the only drug-like treatment that has been shown to work on a continuing basis.[22] In addition, HBOT has been the therapy used on the largest number of patients for the longest period of time (see "MS Patients Band Together for HBOT" on page 50), which means that it is the therapy with the longest period of follow-up results.

The Gottlieb-Neubauer theory, proposing that MS is caused by lack of oxygen, has been supported by research showing that HBOT, which overcomes a lack of oxygen, is an effective treatment method. Established medical circles have come to accept HBOT's effectiveness, although that acceptance was initially slow in coming.

The first sign of this acceptance came in January 1983, when a report on HBOT was published in the prestigious *New England Journal of Medicine* (NEJM). The wording of the report, which came after almost a year of extensive analysis, revision, and review, was cautious. But it did offer a good measure of hope: "These preliminary results [on HBOT] suggest a positive, though transient effect of hyperbaric oxygen on advanced multiple sclerosis (MS) warranting further study."[23] This report's impact on people with MS was electrifying, as they and their families went looking for hyperbaric chambers.[24]

The NEJM report was based on a controlled clinical trial conducted between 1980 and 1982 by Dr. B.H. Fischer, Dr. M. Marks, and Dr. T. Reich at New York University Medical Center. Forty patients with chronic MS were divided randomly into two groups. The experimental group received pure oxygen and the control group received a mixture of 10 percent oxygen and 90 percent nitrogen. Both groups were treated at a pressure of 2.0 atmospheres absolute, but at an effective pressure of only 1.4 atmospheres absolute due to leakage from the masks. Sessions lasted for ninety minutes, once a day, for a total of twenty exposures. (For information on the terms used in hyperbaric medicine, see "The Language of HBOT and of Research" on page 7.)

The investigators discovered that 12 of the 17 patients (70 percent) who received HBOT saw their symptoms improve. (Three of the 20 patients in this group dropped out of the study before it was completed.) But in the control group of patients who inhaled the equivalent of room air under pressure, just 1 in 20 (5 percent) improved.

Of the persons in this study who benefited from HBOT, 7 had short-term relief and 5 had long-lasting relief of MS symptoms. Those with less severe forms of the disease experienced more favorable and prolonged responses.

After one year of followup, deterioration was found in only 2 of the patients (12 percent) who had received pure oxygen, compared with 11 patients (55 percent) in the control group.[25]

A number of studies have criticized HBOT as a treatment for MS. In reviewing many of these studies, Dr. Neubauer believes there were a number of factors that were either not considered or inappropriate. For example, inappropriate pressures were used, patients had advanced MS, and not enough treatments were given. Interestingly enough, one of the authors of a negative report actually went on to open a hyperbaric center in Great Britain specifically to treat MS.

In 1984, Dr. Neubauer learned that more than 10,000 MS patients in fourteen countries had been treated with HBOT. In discussions with his colleagues, he found that the majority of these patients (70 percent) showed improvement in brain and bowel-bladder function, and lessening of muscular spasticity and other systemic disorders brought on by the disease. Objective improvement, or improvement that could be measured, occurred in about 25 percent of the patients. Subjective improvement, or improvement that was noted by the doctor or the patient but is difficult to measure, occurred in about 45 percent of the patients. There was also a marked absence of deterioration and few relapses among patients who participated in a periodic HBOT booster program.

In a double-blind, placebo-controlled 1986 study conducted by Dr. T. Yamada and colleagues in Japan, it was reported that all MS patients treated with HBOT, even for short durations, showed objective improvement. The investigators concluded that long-term HBOT treatment led to a very significant decrease in the number of relapses.[26]

The cases of another 600 MS patients who had been treated with HBOT were reported on by Dr. Neubauer at a hyperbaric medicine conference. Some of these patients stopped receiving HBOT because of cost considerations, or because travel to and from the hyperbaric facility was inconvenient. Others continued to receive treatment. There were significant objective improvements, as well as a reduction in the number of relapses, for those patients who continued HBOT compared with those who did not.

One group that funded extensive research into MS and HBOT was Action for Research into Multiple Sclerosis (ARMS). (See "MS Patients Band Together for HBOT" on page 50.) The results of one ARMS study were published in 1989. This two-year study, conducted by researchers from Ninewells Medical School at the University of Dundee in Scotland, involved 128 HBOT-treated MS pa-

MS Patients Band Together for HBOT

A deeply ingrained desire for self-help has arisen out of the ever-present frustrations experienced by MS patients. Because MS can cause speech difficulties and a lack of physical coordination, people with the disease are often looked upon in a condescending way. Also, many MS patients strive to be involved in finding ways to treat the disease. These patients will often go to any length to find a treatment or cure. Unfortunately, this frequently leads to them being taken advantage of by those who would offer false hope.

In response to these concerns, British MS patients and relatives of patients formed Action for Research into Multiple Sclerosis (ARMS). This group, established in 1974, explored the gaps in medicine's knowledge of the cause, diagnosis, treatment, prevention, and cure of MS. ARMS concluded that HBOT was one of the best ways to keep the disease under control.

ARMS—which, sadly, has gone out of business for lack of funding—looked at all aspects of MS. It offered individual therapy, membership in a network of therapy groups, and a round-the-clock telephone counseling service. As a legacy to MS research, the group left a wealth of useful information, including health, sociological, and psychological profiles on up to 10,000 MS patients, most of whom have been treated with HBOT since 1983.

But the group's greatest achievement was in the development of patient-managed research and therapy programs. In the beginning, ARMS received poor cooperation from the British medical community. Therefore, the group raised its own funds for research into promising new areas that were not receiving adequate support. One of those areas was HBOT.

In 1982, after much study of medical journals, a London lecture on HBOT by Dr. Neubauer, and interviews with other supporters of HBOT in the medical community, ARMS began to set up hyperbaric centers for the benefit of its members. Eventually, there were sixty-three ARMS therapy centers and support groups strategically located around Great Britain, from Shetland in the north to the small island of Jersey in the south. Each center has become a self-sufficient organization, and has provided aid for more than 12,000 patients. This is the largest group of MS patients that has ever been treated with HBOT, and the long-term results of these case studies are becoming available.

What researchers who have looked at this data have found is that while HBOT is not a cure, it has favorably altered the course of these patients' illnesses, just as Dr. Neubauer had predicted in 1978. Many patients treated at centers established by ARMS have stopped experiencing relapses, and some have exhibited near-permanent remissions with continued maintenance treatments. The most significant benefits are in improved balance, muscle control, vision, speech, and sensory perception, and in control of incontinence. This course of treatment—and it does require a long-term commitment by each patient—has enabled patients to lead more normal lives. The notable part of the program is that the centers are operated by the patients themselves, which means that patients who cannot pay for treatment are not turned away.

tients who were compared with an equal number of untreated controls. Seventy percent of the treated MS patients either did not deteriorate, had their conditions stabilize, or showed small improvements.[27]

Behind the studies and statistics are the improvements in daily life experienced by many MS patients who receive HBOT. One Massachusetts woman had been disabled by the disease—she could barely stand and needed a battery-powered cart to move around. She went to Dr. Neubauer's clinic in Florida for help. After her third hour of treatment, she "felt absolutely wonderful and asked my son to get my crutches out of the closet where they were stored. I got up out of my cart and walked around and was astounded at my progress; it was happening that quickly."

When the patient returned to her home, she continued taking HBOT treatments at a hyperbaric center in Pennsylvania. "When I wake up in the morning, I have a very positive, energetic feeling," she said. "I don't in any way see this HBO treatment as being a cure for MS, though. If I hold the line at this point, that's terrific. If I slow down the process of deterioration, that's terrific too, as far as I'm concerned."[28]

As we've seen, HBOT is not a cure for MS. But it has proven to be an effective therapy. It has shown an ability to favorably alter the outcome of the disease. HBOT should be continued in regular, long-term treatments, especially when MS has caused dysfunctions in the part of the brain called the cerebellum, and loss of bowel and bladder control.

For best results, HBOT treatment of MS should be started as early as possible following diagnosis. As with any other illness, MS becomes more difficult to control as the disease process continues. Oxygen cannot and does not reverse plaque formation, and functions best before there has been a consolidation of plaque.

Under an MS treatment plan outlined by Dr. Neubauer,[29] a monoplace chamber is used. The patient receives four one-hour treatments at 1.25 atmospheres absolute, followed by eight treatments at 1.5 atmospheres absolute. Treatments are given once or twice a day. The doctor and patient work closely together to determine which pressure works best for that patient. If there are no positive results, the pressure may be increased up to 1.75 and then up to 2.0 atmospheres absolute, but this is rare. Usually improvement occurs after twenty treatments. Even so, it is important to remember that since the effects of HBOT are cumulative, improvement may not take place until two or three weeks after cessation of treatment.

While the average series of treatments consists of twenty sessions, treatment should continue as long as the patient shows progress. Some patients required as many as eighty exposures in the initial series before stabilization and maximum improvement were achieved, although some improvement may have been made before then. An accurate evaluation of any therapy for MS, including HBOT, cannot be made for at least one to two years.

HBOT can also be used to maintain a remission through the use of from one or two sessions a week, to one or two sessions a month. A twenty-session treatment is given on an annual basis.

Other therapies should be given in conjunction with HBOT. Appropriate therapies include speech and occupational therapies, and massage. Psychotherapy with biofeedback can help the patient's emotional well-being.

In this chapter, we have seen how, in the belief of Dr. Neubauer and Dr. Gottlieb, MS is essentially a circulatory problem linked to a lack of oxygen in the body's tissues. We have also seen how HBOT can overcome this lack of oxygen to help halt the progress of this disease. Unfortunately, this belief is shared by neither a majority of American doctors nor by many MS organizations. Thus, only a handful of hyperbaric centers in the United States will treat MS. Just as insulin injections do not cure diabetes, HBOT does not cure MS. Rather, HBOT provides a significant chance for control and stabilization of MS, as insulin does for diabetes. We hope that a better understanding of this disease on the part of both doctors and patients will encourage more centers to offer MS patients this important treatment. In the next chapter, we'll see how HBOT works in one of its most accepted uses—the treatment of difficult wounds.

CHAPTER 5

Using HBOT to Treat Difficult Wounds

In October 1987, America's attention became riveted on Midland, Texas, where 18-month-old Jessica McClure was trapped twenty-two feet underground after falling into a well. Finally, after two days of digging, Jessica was rescued and rushed to the local hospital. While no bones had been broken, the doctors who treated Jessica feared they might have to amputate the toddler's right foot, as the foot's circulation had been badly impaired. Fortunately, Jessica was not immediately operated on, but was first given HBOT to help improve her circulation and to make it clear how much tissue could be saved. The combination of hyperbaric oxygen and surgery worked. Jessica's little toe was amputated, but her foot was saved, making the toddler one of the world's most famous HBOT patients at the time.

The most common, and often most dramatic, use of HBOT is in the treatment of serious wounds. Each year, Americans make about 25 million visits to emergency rooms because of injuries caused by everything from car accidents to falls to acts of violence. Many of the most severe injuries cause equally severe blood-circulation problems, which in turn bring on oxygen starvation in the body's tissues. Such underoxygenation can disrupt the body's normal functioning almost as much as the actual injuries themselves. HBOT can help patients with severe injuries because of its ability to overcome underoxygenation.

In this chapter, we'll first see why some wounds tend to heal slowly. We'll then discuss how HBOT can be used to help treat such wounds. Burns are covered in Chapter 7. Wounds that affect bones are covered in Chapter 8. Surface wounds caused by various blood-vessel disorders and by diseases such as diabetes are called skin ulcers, and are covered in Chapter 9, as are wounds caused by radiation treatment and skin surgery. (See Appendix A for information on contacting hyperbaric oxygen facilities.)

WHAT MAKES A WOUND DIFFICULT?

In conventional medical practice, HBOT is most widely used to help heal difficult wounds. But before we can look at how this therapy is employed, we must first discuss what makes a wound difficult.

Our first question is, "What is a wound?" A wound is any disruption in the body's tissues. It is often associated with the loss of skin (and underlying tissue), muscle, or bone. Many wounds heal without much medical intervention. Others do not heal, nor do they respond to treatment as expected. The latter wounds are referred to as "difficult," "problem," or "nonhealing" wounds.

Our second question is, "What makes a wound difficult?" Wounds become difficult to treat for several reasons. Sometimes, there is a lack of oxygen in the tissues due to a disruption in the blood supply. This disruption arises after the blood that generally flows from a wound starts to clot. Such clotting interferes with the circulation in the wound area by blocking the blood vessels. Such blockages reduce the area's oxygen supply and prevent removal of wastes produced by the cells. Toxic materials accumulate, and the tissues begin poisoning themselves with their own waste.[1] Certain medical conditions, such as diabetes and collagen vascular disorders, can also cause problems with the body's normal repair processes. That can result in difficulty with wound healing.

The lack of oxygen in a wound starts a cycle of damage. The affected tissues begin to swell. Even when the circulation is restored, the swelling may persist or get worse. That further cuts off the supply of blood and oxygen to the area, and traps even more waste within the tissues. The oxygen depletion and waste buildup combine to kill cells, and the presence of dead cells, in turn, leads to even more oxygen depletion and waste buildup.

Difficult wounds are also prone to infection, a possibility not to be taken lightly. A lack of oxygen in the tissues can reduce the injured person's defense against infection by decreasing the activity of infection-fighting white blood cells.[2-4] A wound's chances of becoming infected are directly related to how little oxygen there is in the affected tissues.[5] Infection can lead to gangrene, which can make it necessary for at least part of the affected limb to be amputated.[6]

Underoxygenation can also reduce the body's ability to heal the wound, especially since healing tissue needs even more oxygen than does healthy tissue.[7] A lack of oxygen can deactivate the cells that produce granulation tissue, the tissue that covers a wound before the new skin grows. It can also interfere with the production of collagen, the basic building material of which new skin is made, and any collagen that is produced is likely to be of poor quality.[8-11]

The creation of capillaries, the tiny blood vessels that connect arteries to veins, requires both collagen and oxygen.[12,13] If either is lacking, new capillaries cannot be created, and wound healing cannot occur. Thus, a lack of oxygen in the wounded tissues can interfere with the entire wound healing process.[14]

Another question we have to ask is, "Can a wound exist even if there is no external bleeding?" The answer is, "Yes." *Compartment syndrome* is a condition caused by inward pressure on an artery. This pressure has the same effect as a blood vessel blockage—it causes a reduction in blood supply that, in turn, produces oxygen depletion and swelling. As the swelling increases, the fluid pressure can become so severe that it brings about a partial or complete collapse of the capillary circulation within the affected tissues. If this collapse occurs, gangrene—tissue death—can set in. Therefore, compartment syndrome can carry with it a considerable risk of amputation.[15,16] It can even result in a permanent contraction of the affected hand or foot. Unfortunately, such permanent deformities are not reversed by HBOT.

HBOT AND THE HEALING OF DIFFICULT WOUNDS

As we've seen, a lack of oxygen can make it difficult for a wound to heal. That makes HBOT an important part of a total wound-healing treatment plan. We'll first see how HBOT helps heal wounds. We'll then take a look at how doctors at a distinguished trauma center in Belgium employ HBOT in their work.

How HBOT Helps Heal Wounds

HBOT is the best way of increasing the oxygen content of underoxygenated tissues.[17-21] It can reduce swelling by constricting blood vessels. At the same time HBOT can put more oxygen in the body's fluids, and thus is able to deliver more oxygen to underoxygenated tissues.[22,23] The constricted blood vessels keep excess fluid out of the wounded area, which allows nutrients to reach the affected tissues and waste products to be carried away. That keeps cells from dying. At the same time, the extra oxygen in the body's fluids means that, even with less blood flowing into the area, the wounded tissues get the oxygen they need to begin the healing process. Thus, the use of HBOT is a very valuable way of treating difficult wounds.[24-27]

The use of HBOT can provide various benefits in the treatment of difficult wounds:

• *It makes it easy to see what tissue must be removed.* When HBOT is given, a very clear line of demarcation develops between tissue which is beyond repair and that which can be saved.[28] This demarcation makes it easier for the doctor to see what tissue must be removed.

- *It lessens the chance of infection.* Underoxygenation makes a wound more susceptible to infection, which slows the rate of healing.[29-31] Swelling reduces the number of white blood cells and other infection fighters that can reach the affected tissues, and those cells that do find their way to the area cannot act very effectively without oxygen. Also, some of the most dangerous microbes in wounds are anaerobic, which means that they thrive in the absence of oxygen. HBOT can help counteract infection indirectly by providing the white blood cells with the oxygen they need. It can also act directly by killing anaerobic organisms, stopping their multiplication, and neutralizing the toxins that some of them produce.[32,33] HBOT also helps antibiotics such as sulfa drugs work more effectively.[34-38] (For more information on HBOT and infection, see Chapter 6.)

- *It encourages the growth of new tissue.* The extra oxygen provided by HBOT helps the body create the different types of tissues needed in wound healing. Oxygen is essential in the creation of granulation tissue, the pink, fleshy tissue that first grows over a healing wound.[39] Granulation tissue can be seen within seven to ten days of starting a patient on HBOT. By thirty days, this tissue becomes densely supplied with blood vessels.[40] Oxygen also promotes the growth of collagen, the material of which skin and connective tissue are formed. Collagen, in turn, forms the bed on which new capillaries are created. Therefore, the more collagen is produced, the more quickly the new skin's blood supply is created.

- *It encourages bone repair.* Bone repair depends on the action of osteoclasts, cells that dispose of dead bone, and osteoblasts, cells that create new bone. In turn, these cells depend on a rich supply of oxygen, which is best supplied by HBOT. (For more information on HBOT and bone repair, see Chapter 8.)

HBOT's effectiveness in minimizing tissue death, reducing swelling, and promoting healing has been proven in the laboratory.[41-43] It has also been proven in case studies (for information on research terms, see "The Language of HBOT and of Research" on page 7). For example, seven teams of researchers published reports in English-language medical journals about the successful use of HBOT for crush injuries and compartment syndrome. All the patients—including ninety-three trauma cases—showed extensive benefits.[44-50] And a series of reports from the Eastern European medical literature, 634 cases in all, also attested to the benefits of HBOT.[51]

In two reports from the 1980s, a total of 13 patients who had suffered acute blood loss from leg wounds found great advantages in HBOT. The injuries were caused by shrapnel wounds, auto accidents, and other crush traumas. In all of the cases, there was a delay of almost twelve hours from the time of accident to the time of surgery. Some of the cases were complicated by the existence of severe infection and compound fractures (see "Different Types of Fractures" on page 85), with associated nerve and blood-vessel damage. In four cases, the limbs were saved. In two other cases, the use of HBOT allowed doctors to perform amputations lower down on the leg than would have been required had HBOT not been used. Without HBOT, all of the patients would have had to undergo extensive amputations.[52,53] The earlier and more frequently HBOT is used, the more likely it is that severely injured body parts will be saved.[54-56]

One Trauma Center's Use of HBOT

One of the most respected trauma surgery units in the world is the Department of Microsurgery at the University of Liege Hospital in Belgium. HBOT plays an important part in the department's work. For example, between 1978 and 1989, this unit used HBOT in the treatment of 390 patients suffering from serious limb wounds. These were the worst kind of injuries, with significant tissue destruction, total lack of blood vessel supply, skin and muscle death, open fractures, contaminated wounds, compartment syndrome, and limb loss. Most of the wounds involved the legs (58 percent), followed by the arms (26 percent), the abdomen (11 percent), the chest (3 percent), and the head (2 percent). Vehicular injuries accounted for 60 percent of the cases, while 40 percent resulted from domestic or industrial causes. Of those people suffering from vehicular injury, 60 percent were under forty years of age. Most of the patients were men.[57]

More than 85 percent of these patients underwent surgery before receiving HBOT. Surgical procedures included cleaning wounds of dirt and dead tissue, decompressing compartment syndromes, and stabilizing fractures, in addition to repairing muscles, blood vessels, and nerves. Often, skin grafts were necessary. Frequently, patients had to return to the operating room for dressing changes and additional tissue removal under anesthesia.

The basic HBOT procedure was adapted to each individual's special needs. But usually, treatment was given in monoplace chambers, with pressure at 3.0 atmospheres absolute for sixty minutes (see "The Language of HBOT and of Research" on page 7). The first session was usually performed immediately following surgery, and treatment was repeated every eight hours for the first day and a half. The patients then underwent two sessions daily for the following two days, and one session daily for up to four days. In some cases, HBOT sessions were necessary for two or three more weeks because of the nature of the injuries involved. Each patient received between three and forty-five sessions, with a mean average of twelve sessions. Only one of the patients treated with HBOT developed gas gangrene (see Chapter 6).

HBOT's benefits were noted by the medical staff, the most visibly obvious benefit being the reduction in cyanosis, or blueness of the tissues caused by lack of oxygen.[58] The Liege doctors were convinced that HBOT helped them heal difficult wounds and save reattached limbs that would otherwise have not been healed or saved. (See "Using HBOT to Help Save Body Parts".)

One of the Liege cases is a particularly powerful example of how HBOT can help a patient to overcome a serious injury. In this case, a police officer, twenty-five years old, suffered numerous severe injuries in an automobile accident. These injuries included a crushed and severed left foot and ankle. The patient was in serious shock when he was brought to the emergency room, where he received intravenous fluids, blood transfusions, and antibiotics. He was then transferred to an operating room for an attempted reattachment of his foot.

The surgery lasted for fifteen hours. It involved recreating the lower tibia, the large bone in the lower leg, from bone taken elsewhere from the patient's body. The doctors also had to bypass arteries and veins; suture nerves, tendons, and muscles; graft skin; and attach connective tissue.

Following this extensive surgery, the patient received a total of twenty-five HBOT treatments to promote healing of the reattached tissues. The wounds healed gradually, and the patient returned to the operating room only for dressing changes and removal of dead skin. One month later, he was released with his left foot and ankle fully reattached and intact. Two further surgeries were needed to correct bone problems.

The treatment was successful. The patient recovered his ability to walk normally. Over time, he also regained full nerve sensibility in his foot. The doctors who treated him attributed his recovery to their vigorous use of HBOT. Excellent healing after all of this surgery was an astonishing testimonial to the beneficial qualities of hyperbaric oxygen.[59]

The Liege treatment plan calls for one HBOT session, at 3.0 atmospheres absolute, immediately following surgery. A second treatment should be given eight hours after surgery, a third after sixteen hours, and then twice a day for two more days. After that, HBOT should be given once a day for a period ranging from three days to three weeks or

Using HBOT to Help Save Body Parts

Emergency room personnel see hundreds of cases of severed body parts each year, mostly fingers lost in industrial accidents and feet or legs lost in motor vehicle accidents. At one time, doctors could only care for the wounds and fit the patients with prostheses. But now, thanks to improved surgical techniques and the use of HBOT, many of these patients are having major body parts successfully reattached.

One of the most important factors in the success of a limb replant is the time period between injury and repair. A severed limb kept at room temperature must be reattached within six hours, or the procedure will not work. There are two ways of prolonging limb life: keeping the limb cold or using HBOT. HBOT can keep the limb alive for up to thirty-six hours following the injury.

A total limb transplant requires various types of surgical procedures. Plastic and reconstructive surgery are needed in cases where large areas of skin and bone are torn away. When local tissue is not available, the surgeon can take transplants from other areas of the patient's body. In the case of an ear or a nose, the surgeon borrows cartilage, usually from the patient's ribs, to create a new part. Moving body parts from one place to another, such as using a toe in place of a finger, is another option.

The most critical reattachments are those of the blood vessels and nerves. These connections are done via microsurgery, in which the surgeon uses a microscope and sutures thinner than a human hair to connect the severed structures. Nerves are the most difficult organs to reattach, since each nerve may have many thousands of individual nerve fibers within it.

HBOT is critically important after surgery because it helps insure good oxygenation through the reattached part, which lessens the chances of blood clot formation. HBOT also helps put extra oxygen into the affected tissues, which need a good supply of oxygen in order for healing to take place.

The use of mechanical, or bionic, body parts is a main-

stay of television and movies. But bionics represents hard-
ware. It is the goal of most surgeons to successfully reattach a patient's own severed limb. HBOT has helped make
that goal a reality for many patients.

longer, depending on the extent of the injuries and the
presence of any complications. HBOT should be used
along with physical therapy to help the patient recover as
full a range of motion and function as possible.

In this chapter, we've seen how HBOT can assist people
to recover from serious injuries, including the loss of
limbs, by improving circulation and providing wounded
tissues with much-needed oxygen. In the next chapter,
we'll see how HBOT can help people recover from infection, including gas gangrene, a potentially fatal wound infection.

CHAPTER 6

Using HBOT to Treat Infections

In Florida, 56-year-old Gerald R. suffers severe scratches to both hands while cleaning out a rose bed. He goes to the emergency room and is treated with antiseptics, but not antibiotics. Within forty-eight hours, his hands are hot and tender, and the scratches are oozing. Antibiotics are given, and cultures eventually reveal a serious strep infection. Meanwhile, the wounds open up, and Gerald is admitted to the hospital. His wounds are thoroughly cleaned and he is put on intravenous antibiotics, but his condition does not improve. Gerald's doctors, worried that he might lose his hands, add HBOT to his treatment plan. After the fourth treatment, the oozing and swelling are reduced, and Gerald feels better. After the twentieth treatment, Gerald's hands are all but healed, and his doctors are pleased at his response to HBOT.

Throughout the course of human history, infection has been one of the leading causes of death. Infectious diseases such as bubonic plague have decimated civilizations.

Humankind began to win the war on infection with the development of sulfa drugs in the 1930s and penicillin in the 1940s. Since then, many of the world's most dreaded diseases, from cholera to polio, have been conquered. However, there are particularly stubborn infections that have proven hard to subdue, and HBOT has proven itself to be a useful treatment for some of these infections. In this chapter, we will first look at how HBOT helps fight infection. We will then see how this therapy has been used to treat specific infections. (See Appendix A for information on contacting hyperbaric oxygen facilities.)

FIGHTING INFECTION WITH HBOT

Oxygen acts as a potent antibiotic. Oxygen dissolved in the blood improves the ability of special scavenger white blood cells, called phagocytes, to rid the body of bacteria and other foreign proteins. Since HBOT forces oxygen into the body's tissues, it has a distinct antimicrobial effect that is equal to or better than that of numerous antibiotics. HBOT may also enhance the actions of certain antibiotics and thereby increase their effectiveness in overcoming infections.

HBOT helps fight all microorganisms, but especially those that thrive in the absence of oxygen. These are called *anaerobic* organisms. Microorganisms that thrive in the presence of oxygen are called *aerobic* organisms. There is evidence that HBOT, because of its immune system-enhancing effects, can help the body fight these microbes, too.[1–10]

GAS GANGRENE AND HBOT

Gas gangrene is a painful condition in which the body's soft tissues are destroyed by toxins produced by bacteria. It is usually caused by a microbe called *Clostridium perfringens,* which is implicated in 80 to 90 percent of all cases of gas gangrene. This disease is usually associated with surgery or with massive trauma, such as that found on the battlefield or following car accidents. Gas gangrene is characterized by profound blood poisoning, extensive swelling, massive death of tissue, and the production of gas in the affected areas. Initial symptoms include pain and tenderness in the wound area, mild fever, and rapid heartbeat. The patient may develop life-threatening anemia, kidney failure, jaundice, brain dysfunction, and heart toxicity. About 1,100 Americans die of gas gangrene each year.

Clostridium perfringens is an anaerobic bacterium, the kind that thrives in the absence of oxygen. What happens in gas gangrene is that the initial injury results in hypoxia, or a lack of oxygen in the tissues. The bacteria thrive under these conditions, and produce toxins that cause swelling. The swelling further diminishes the supply of both blood and oxygen to the area. That keeps the immune system from functioning properly, which in turn allows the disease to spread and produce even more toxins. (Clostridium toxin is very virulent. It has been estimated that a pint of this toxin could kill a substantial portion of the world's population.) It all happens so quickly that the body cannot fight the spread of the disease. As a result, the patient can become gravely ill within twelve hours.

While antibiotics and surgery are the main forms of treatment for gas gangrene, HBOT has been shown to be a significant adjunct. HBOT works against the clostridia bacteria by killing the organisms and deactivating the toxins. That serves to counteract the low-oxygen environment in which the bacteria thrive. The high levels of oxygen, in turn, lead to the death or inactivation of the microbes. However, dead tissue creates toxins that can keep HBOT from doing its job, which is why surgery is often necessary for HBOT to work most effectively. Once the dead tissue is removed, the oxygen can act freely against the bacteria.[11–16]

Using surgery and HBOT together helps both the patient and the doctor. HBOT's ability to neutralize the clostridium toxin means less tissue death. Also, HBOT clarifies the line between live tissue and dead tissue. When a person infected with clostridia is treated with HBOT, a clear distinction develops within hours between that tissue which must be cut out and that which can be saved. In this way, both the number and the extent of amputations can be reduced. Moreover, HBOT can save lives because it decreases the extent of surgery that needs to be performed on gravely ill patients, for whom surgery carries considerable risk.

Such a treatment program is strengthened by the addition of antibiotics. A three-part plan that employs surgery, HBOT, and antibiotics causes survival rates to increase from 50 percent for antibiotics together alone, and 80 percent for surgery plus HBOT, to up to 95 percent for all three combined.[17,18]

Extensive evidence in the medical literature supports the use of HBOT as part of an overall treatment plan for gas gangrene. More than 4,000 cases of gas gangrene treated with HBOT have been reported in medical journals. Here are conclusions taken from just a few of these studies:

- In one study, there was a survival rate of 88.3 percent among 248 patients who received HBOT.[19]

- A study by Dr. M.E. Ellis and Dr. B.K. Mandal analyzed the cases of 58 patients who had failed to respond to antibiotics and surgery, and who were considered to have poor prognoses. After these patients received HBOT, there was a survival rate of 84 percent. Survivors showed a marked improvement in their conditions.[20]

- In another study of 139 patients treated with HBOT, there was a survival rate of 70 percent. Eighty percent of the survivors were able to avoid amputations (some patients had more than one limb involved).[21]

Treatment for gas gangrene should include surgery, antibiotics, and HBOT. (There is a gas gangrene antitoxin, but this produces adverse reactions in about 10 percent of the patients who receive it.) The oxygen should be administered at 3.0 atmospheres absolute[22] (see "The Language of HBOT and of Research" on page 7) in ninety-minute sessions. These sessions should be given at least twice a day until the patient improves, which may require up to twelve treatments. However, only three or four sessions are usually required, in conjunction with surgery and antibiotics as needed.

LYME DISEASE AND HBOT

Lyme disease is a tick-borne illness with a wide array of symptoms. It is named for the town of Old Lyme, Connecticut, where it was first described in 1975. While cases have been reported throughout the country, the disease is most prevalent in the Northeast and upper Midwest. It is similar to other tick-borne diseases that have been recognized in Europe for more than 100 years.

Lyme disease is caused by a corkscrew-shaped bacterium called a spirochete, usually *Borrelia burgdorferi.* The spirochete is carried by the deer tick, a tiny creature that in the adult stage is about the size of a sesame seed. These ticks pick up the disease from various animal hosts, especially mice, before passing it on to human beings. Because the tick is so small, bites often go unnoticed.

The first sign of Lyme disease is a usually painless skin rash called *erythema migrans* at or near the site of the bite. This rash, which generally has a bull's-eye appearance, develops within a week after the bite occurs and usually lasts a few days, although in rare cases it may last a month or more. The rash is a positive sign of Lyme disease, even when blood tests are negative. Unfortunately, 25 percent or more of the people who develop Lyme disease do not develop the rash. Others may not notice the rash before it disappears.

If not promptly and properly treated, Lyme disease can produce the following conditions:

- Nervous-system problems, including inflammation either of the membranes covering the brain and spinal cord (meningitis) or of the brain itself (encephalitis). Some patients may develop confusion, memory loss, and emotional difficulties.

- Heart problems, including inflammation of the heart (myocarditis) and heart block, an abnormal slowing of the heartbeat.

- Joint problems, usually arthritis of the larger joints such as the knee.

- Various other problems, including fever, fatigue, headache, and muscle pain.

Lyme disease can be very difficult to identify, especially if the patient does not develop or notice the characteristic rash. One problem is that the symptoms of Lyme disease mimic those of various other diseases, which means it can easily be misdiagnosed and mistreated. Another problem is that the various blood tests used to detect Lyme disease are not always reliable. Two out of three patients do not test positive when they are first diagnosed. Conversely, many patients may test positive for several years after the symptoms disappear.

Lyme disease has been difficult to treat. If caught early, oral antibiotics can usually cure the patient. However, if the disease is not detected early, the body's own cells tend to protect the Lyme spirochete against antibiotics. Thus, even when very strong drugs are used, the spirochete may not be completely destroyed. At this stage, antibiotics are given intravenously. Some patients are cured with intravenous antibiotics, but many patients have received this treatment for several years without relief.

Studies suggest that HBOT works against Lyme disease by attacking the spirochete itself.[23–25] Pure oxygen inhaled at ground-level pressures does not appear to affect the spirochete because not enough oxygen can penetrate the body's cells under these conditions. (For information on atmospheric pressure, see "The Language of HBOT and of Research" on page 7.) However, HBOT can force oxygen into the body's cells, where it can act against the Lyme spirochete.

Preliminary evidence of HBOT's effectiveness against Lyme disease in humans was provided by a pilot study conducted by Dr. William Fife and Dr. Donald Freeman at Texas A&M University.[26] In this study, 40 patients were treated with HBOT at a pressure of 2.36 atmospheres absolute once or twice a day, five days a week, for from one to four weeks. Some patients continued antibiotic therapy while taking HBOT. Others did not.

In response to treatment, all of the patients developed a sudden, passing fever called a Jarisch-Herxheimer reaction, a reaction that also often appears during aggressive antibiotic therapy for Lyme disease. This reaction tended to diminish over two or three weeks. Some patients felt relief of symptoms during the course of treatment. Others did not, but showed improvement a few weeks after the treatments ended. In all but 2 cases, any improvements that were reported continued after the patients left the study, even if they did not resume antibiotic treatment. Improvements included elimination of mental confusion and depression, relief of pain, and increased energy. In a number of cases, the patients still suffered minor Lyme symptoms after taking HBOT, but usually with nothing near the same severity.

The use of HBOT in the treatment of Lyme disease is a relatively recent development. Therefore, no standard treatment plan yet exists. Nevertheless, the study by Dr. Fife and Dr. Freeman, preliminary as it is, indicates great promise for the use of HBOT in this area. Additional studies are needed.

OTHER INFECTIONS AND HBOT

HBOT can be employed to treat a variety of other infections. Three of those infections are streptococcal infections, leprosy, and actinomycosis.

Streptococcal infections are caused by bacteria in the *Streptococci* family, a large family of bacteria that can cause infections in various parts of the body. One place a streptococcal infection can develop is the skin. The virulence of some of these infections has led to news reports of "flesh-eating bacteria."

Streptococcal infections of the skin can develop after a wound occurs, or can spread to the skin from another site via the bloodstream. In either case, the bacteria secrete digestive enzymes that break down tissue. That accounts for the infection's rapid spread. In deeper tissues, a streptococcal infection can cause *necrotizing fasciitis*, a severe infection of the body's connective tissue, or *myositis*, a muscle infection.

Treatment of a streptococcal infection requires high dosages of intravenous antibiotics, and radical surgery to remove infected tissue. HBOT is useful because, as in the case of gas gangrene, it can increase the effectiveness of antibiotics, show where diseased tissue ends and healthy tissue begins, and provide high levels of oxygen to help in the repair process.

The usual treatment plan uses oxygen given at between 2.4 and 3.0 atmospheres absolute (see "The Language of HBOT and of Research" on page 7) for ninety minutes. If the infection is severe or widespread, the patient is initially given two treatments a day for two or three days until the condition stabilizes. The patient then receives HBOT once a day until the infection is gone and healthy tissue is present. Filling in the defect may require a skin graft, and usually ten HBOT sessions are given after the grafting operation.

Leprosy, also known as Hansen's disease, is a chronic bacterial disease that, contrary to common belief, is not very contagious. It affects mainly the peripheral nerves and the skin, but sometimes spreads to other organs as well. Symptoms include loss of sensation and the development of growths or ulcers in the skin.

Leprosy was the first infectious disease to be treated with HBOT: in 1938, doctors in Brazil gave it to 9 patients, with good results.[27] Two later studies also showed positive results.[28,29]

Antimicrobial therapy for leprosy is very effective, and patients can usually be cured with few residual results. In some cases, the patient must take antibiotics for life. HBOT is effective in situations in which drug resistance develops. It is also helpful in patients who are severely anemic, with low hemoglobin counts, and who must wait until their blood counts improve before beginning antibiotic therapy.

There is no standardized HBOT treatment plan for leprosy.

Actinomycosis, or lumpy jaw, is an infection caused by a bacterium called *Actinomyces israelii*. It mostly occurs among those who work with animals, as both cattle and hogs can transmit the disease to human beings. (However, people cannot transmit the disease to each other.) It can also occur after tooth or tonsil infections. Actinomycosis results in deep, lumpy holes that produce pus. The infection can spread to other parts of the body, including the liver, spine, brain, kidneys, genitals, and spleen.

Because actinomycosis can be a long-term problem that is very slow to heal, some cases do not respond to antibiotics and surgical drainage. In contrast, HBOT has proved to be a superb therapy for this fungal infection.

The *Actinomyces* bacteria is very sensitive to the antibiotics penicillin and clindamycin. About 70 percent of all patients respond to surgery and antibiotics alone. Because of this, few cases have been treated with HBOT. However, HBOT has been shown to be of great value in cases where surgery would be disfiguring and in those patients who do not respond to surgery and antibiotics.

When HBOT is used, actinomycosis is treated with ninety minutes of oxygen at 3.0 atmospheres absolute. Seven sessions are given the first day, two are given the second day, and one treatment a day is given the third and fourth days.[30]

In this chapter, we have seen how HBOT can help fight a number of serious infections. Of all the different types of wounds, burns are among the most prone to infection. In the next chapter, we'll see how HBOT not only combats burn infections, but can help heal the burns themselves.

CHAPTER 7

Using HBOT
to Treat Burns

In Texas, 34-year-old Dominic M., a firefighter, is rushed to the hospital from a fire scene. He has second- and third-degree burns over 60 percent of his body. There was a time when a patient suffering from such severe burns would have almost surely died, or have been left disabled with massive scars. However, thanks to improvements in burn care, including skin grafts and HBOT, patients such as Dominic have a much better chance of surviving their injuries. Dominic does survive. He returns to work—and becomes a father.

Serious burns—which can be caused by chemicals and electricity as well as by fire—can be among the most painful of injuries, and among the most difficult to treat. Each year, some 38,500 Americans are burned badly enough to require skin grafts for survival. There are also 80,000 burn victims each year who don't need skin transplants but who do need medical assistance. HBOT can help burn patients heal faster with fewer complications. (See Chapter 5 for information on HBOT and other types of difficult wounds, and Appendix A for a list of hyperbaric oxygen facilities.)

WHY ARE SOME BURNS SO HARD TO TREAT?

Burns range in severity from first degree to third degree. In a *first-degree burn*, only the top layer of skin is involved.

The skin is red but unbroken, and there is no danger of infection. In a *second-degree burn*, deeper skin layers are involved. The skin is reddened and blistered. Often, there is a massive loss of fluid, and the resulting dehydration may deepen the wound. In a *third-degree burn*, the entire thickness of skin is involved. The skin may be charred, and there may be little pain initially because of the loss of nerve endings in the affected skin area.

The severity of a burn is also judged by how extensive it is. Small burns cover up to 15 percent of the body's surface area. Moderate burns cover 15 to 49 percent, large burns cover 50 to 69 percent, while massive burns cover 70 percent or more of the body's surface. Both the degree and the extent of a burn must be taken into account when deciding how severe a burn is. In the case of a first-degree burn, professional medical attention is not needed unless the burn covers a large area of skin. Both second- and third-degree burns require emergency medical treatment, especially if they cover more than 10 percent of the body, since such burns can easily lead to shock. Serious burns can also become infected.

In order for a burn to heal properly, it is very important for the burned area to develop new skin rapidly and cleanly. Sometimes, the wound is so extensive that skin grafts—either skin taken from elsewhere on the patient or an artificial skin product—have to be used (see Chapter 9). At other times, the body can create new skin itself. The body's ability to do so depends upon four factors:[1]

• The total number of skin cells surviving the injury

• The migration of viable cells from healthy areas into the wound

• The ability of both the surviving and the migrating cells to reproduce

• The development of new capillaries

USING HBOT IN BURN TREATMENT

A roaring explosion deep in a Japanese coal mine in 1965 is responsible for the accidental discovery that HBOT speeds the healing of burns while reducing infection. Many of the miners caught in the blast were overcome by carbon monoxide, and so were rushed to the nearby hospital's hyperbaric chamber. (See Chapter 10 for information on HBOT and carbon monoxide poisoning.) A few days later, the doctors noted a remarkable coincidence. The burns of those patients affected by carbon monoxide poisoning were healing faster, and with fewer infections, than those of the other miners. The only difference in treatment was that the better-healing group had been in the hyperbaric chamber.[2]

The use of HBOT within the first twenty-four hours after the injury can promote the conditions needed for the body to recover from a severe burn. It can help wounded cells survive by constricting blood vessels in the area. This means that less fluid is lost, so that wounded cells do not dry out and die. HBOT can also supply the wound with extra oxygen, despite the blood-vessel constriction. That's because HBOT forces oxygen not only into the red blood cells, the part of the blood that normally carries oxygen, but into the blood plasma and other body fluids. This extra oxygen also helps wounded cells to survive, and can help cells to reproduce. And by contributing to the establishment of a new network of capillaries, the tiny blood vessels that connect arteries to veins, HBOT can cause cells from healthy areas to migrate into the wound.

There is evidence that HBOT can also help burn patients by:

- Preventing burn shock, or circulatory failure produced by massive fluid loss

- Inhibiting wound infection, both by helping to support the body's infection-fighting white blood cells and by helping to increase the effectiveness of any antibiotics that are given (see Chapter 6)

- Aiding in the survival of skin grafts and flaps, and in the growth of new skin
- Reducing the need for fluids
- Reducing the rate of complications
- Helping the patient cope with other serious problems that often accompany burns, such as smoke inhalation and carbon monoxide poisoning (see Chapter 10)

All of these factors help to speed healing and to increase the survival rate among burn patients. One study showed that the hospitalization and mortality rates among severely burned patients who received HBOT were reduced by a third, compared with the rates of those patients who did not receive hyperbaric oxygen. The HBOT-treated patients also required one-third less fluid replacement.[3]

HBOT usefulness in aiding burn recovery has been shown in animal studies.[4] A 1977 rabbit study showed that healing occurred 30 percent faster when HBOT was used.[5] A study done with rats showed similar results.[6] In 1978, researchers found that HBOT helped bring about spontaneous healing in guinea pigs. It also helped skin grafts become well established, regardless of the depth of the burn and whether it was second or third degree in extent.[7] In 1985, another guinea pig study showed that the use of HBOT resulted in better healing.[8]

A 1974 study by Dr. G.B. Hart and colleagues looked at 191 human burn patients. The results showed decreases in healing time, complication rate, and mortality rate for patients who were treated with HBOT within the first twenty-four hours after the injury. The time required for healing was related directly to the number of burns and the percentage of body surface involved. The researchers concluded that while HBOT is not a cure-all for burn patients, it can play a significant role in a total burn-treatment program.[9]

Other parts of a burn-treatment program include:

- Wound cleansing
- Debridement, or removal of dead skin
- Use of intravenous fluids to counteract fluid loss
- Treatment of shock
- Treatment of lung problems caused by smoke inhalation or exposure to toxins, such as carbon monoxide
- Administration of tetanus booster or vaccine, depending on the patient's last immunization

The use of appropriate splints and pressure garments can help preserve appearance and function as the wounds heal. Proper body positioning during the healing process and the movement of affected joints can help prevent contractures, which can cause deformities and hinder the patient's range of motion.

Burn expert and plastic surgeon Dr. Richard Grossman developed an HBOT treatment program at Sherman Oaks Community Hospital in Sherman Oaks, California, in which HBOT is given within four hours of the patient's admission to the burn unit. The pressure used is between 2.0 and 2.5 atmospheres absolute, with the length of time to be decided by the hyperbaricist. (For more information on HBOT terminology, see "The Language of HBOT and of Research" on page 7.) Dr. Grossman also uses HBOT both before and after operating on burn patients.[10]

We have seen that HBOT is a useful part of an overall treatment program for burns, in part by helping to prevent the complications that so often accompany serious burns. This therapy can also help people who have developed complications resulting from other types of injuries. In the next chapter, we will discuss how HBOT can help patients who suffer from the complications that sometimes follow bone injuries.

CHAPTER 8

Using HBOT
to Treat Bone Disorders

In Texas, 24-year-old Maria M., a professional violinist, develops a bone infection in the third finger of her left hand after injuries sustained in a dune buggy accident. Eighteen months of conventional treatment, including antibiotics and the surgical removal of dead tissue, cannot cure it. Maria is in danger of losing both her finger and her career. She then spends a month undergoing HBOT for two hours each day, and the stubborn infection finally heals. A grateful Maria returns to the hospital where she was treated to give a concert—for the staff of the hyperbaric oxygen facility.

Every day, people from all walks of life suffer bone injuries, from the high school football player making a tackle to the middle-aged motorist involved in a car accident. The majority of these injuries involve fractures of various kinds. For most of the people suffering these injuries, a trip to the emergency room results in a set fracture, and after a month or two of cast and cane, their lives return to normal.

However, some people with bone injuries develop complications that can cause great pain, and in some cases, limb loss. Some of these complications follow fractures, while others can result from other sorts of injuries. In this chapter, we will first see how bone growth can be disrupted by disease, and how HBOT can help stop this disruption. We'll then look at three bone disorders—osteomyelitis, aseptic bone necrosis, and fracture nonunion—and how they can be helped by HBOT. (See Chapter 5 for information on how HBOT can be used to treat other kinds of difficult wounds, and Appendix A for information on contacting hyperbaric oxygen facilities.)

BONE HEALING AND HBOT

A bone has three layers of tissue: a spongy inner layer, a rigid middle layer, and a tough outer layer. Bones are rigid because of the minerals, mainly calcium, that are found in the middle and outer layers. The bones of children contain less calcium than the bones of adults, which means that children's bones are more pliable. In the long bones of the legs and arms, the inner layer is known as the *marrow*, and is the place where red blood cells are formed.

When bone is injured, special cells called *osteoclasts* work to repair the damage. These cells carve paths through bone tissue around the break and cause dead bone to be reabsorbed by the body. Other cells called *osteoblasts* then create new bone. If the osteoclasts don't break down the dead and infected bone, a diseased area of tissue will remain, which will make it very difficult for the bone to heal correctly.

The osteoclasts depend on oxygen for proper functioning. However, injury often results in hypoxia, or a lack of oxygen in the body's tissues. Hypoxia occurs because many small blood vessels are destroyed, which means that oxygen-rich blood cannot reach the injured area. In fact, osteomyelitis, one of the diseases we'll be discussing in this chapter, has been linked to a lack of blood vessels at the site of a bone infection.[1,2]

HBOT helps to heal bone disorders by stimulating both the osteoclasts and the osteoblasts.[3,4] This reinvigoration leads to the reabsorption of dead bone and the creation of new bone. In addition, HBOT stimulates the production of new blood vessels, so that the growing bone receives a steady supply of nutrients, including oxygen. This blood-vessel network does two other things: it helps support the function of the osteoclasts, and it brings infection-fighting white blood cells to the area.

WHEN BONES BECOME INFECTED: OSTEOMYELITIS

Osteomyelitis is a bacterial infection that usually involves both of the outer layers of bone, as well as the inner bone marrow. Staphylococci (staph) bacteria, a common form of bacteria that can cause infections ranging from pimples to meningitis, are often involved.

The germs that cause osteomyelitis can enter the bone during an injury or during surgery. Osteomyelitis is an ever-present hazard following compound fractures (see "Different Types of Fractures" on page 85). It must also be rigorously guarded against whenever the marrow is exposed during bone or joint surgery.

Germs may also reach the bone directly from a nearby infection or indirectly through the bloodstream. The long bones in children and the spinal bones in adults usually are the sites of infection caused by bacteria spreading from other parts of the body.

Osteomyelitis can be either acute or chronic. All cases are initially acute. There may be severe pain, swelling, and redness at the site of the infection, often on the long bone shaft, accompanied by general illness and extremely high fever. Chronic osteomyelitis may follow the acute form or may develop over time, when the acute form is not completly cured by treatment. Its symptoms include bone pain, tenderness, local muscle spasm, and fever. Long-term osteomyelitis may go on for years, with periods of worsening or waning symptoms, in spite of treatment.

Conventional treatment of osteomyelitis includes several weeks of bed rest and antibiotics. Surgery may be necessary to take out dead bone and soft tissue, to fill holes, and to implant artificial devices designed to keep the diseased bones and joints from moving. The term *refractory osteomyelitis* refers to those cases that have failed to heal in spite of adequate surgical and antibiotic therapy.

All bone infections must be treated promptly and vigorously, as they tend to spread to other parts of the body. When this happens, such infections are often difficult to reach and destroy. Even the most minor infections can cause difficulty. For instance, osteomyelitis sometimes occurs after tooth extraction, even when comprehensive antibiotic therapy is used. The dentist and the patient then face an intractable infection of the bone.

Part of the difficulty in treating osteomyelitis lies in the fact that it causes a lack of oxygen in the tissues, and some bone itself has few blood vessels. HBOT, by providing forced oxygenation, helps fight this disease in three ways. First, it helps strengthen the bone cells called osteoclasts that reabsorb dead bone, allowing those osteoclasts to remove bony debris more effectively. Second, HBOT enhances the function of the immune system's white blood cells, since these cells depend on oxygen. In this respect, HBOT is especially effective when used with antibiotics. And third, HBOT helps the body to create new blood vessels. As a result of these three factors, the body is able to get rid of the diseased bone and replace it with healthy bone.

Doctors first discovered HBOT's effectiveness in the treatment of osteomyelitis back in 1968, in studies done with laboratory rats. The animals were cured of bone infections—with symptoms that included sinus infections, abscesses, and bony deterioration—through the use of HBOT alone. No antibiotics were used, and surgery was not performed. The animals in this study were divided into various groups according to the oxygen pressures used. Best results were obtained in the group treated with 2.0 atmospheres absolute for two hours, three times a day

Different Types of Fractures

An injury to a bone in which the tissue of the bone is broken is called a fracture. There are many different fracture classifications, but they generally fall into four basic types— greenstick, simple, comminuted, and compound. In a *greenstick fracture*, the break does not go all the way through the bone and, in fact, looks like a green twig that has been twisted. This fracture often occurs in children, since their bones are more pliable than those of adults. In a *simple fracture*, there is a clean break of the bone with little damage to surrounding tissues and no break in the overlying skin. Such a fracture is usually simple to set and generally involves no complications. In a *comminuted fracture*, the bone is broken in more than two places. Healing of a comminuted fracture is usually slow because the blood supply is interrupted. In a *compound fracture*, the broken end of the bone pierces the overlying skin and can cause considerable tissue damage. This fracture can be difficult to set and carries a risk of infection. And if a bone is already diseased, even normal stress may cause a break. This is called a *pathological fracture*.

Fractures are also classified according to the bone involved. For example, a simple tibial fracture is a simple fracture of the tibia, which is the large bone in the lower leg.

(see "The Language of HBOT and of Research" on page 7). HBOT given before infections developed did not prevent infections from taking hold. Therefore, the researchers concluded that HBOT works in cases of established osteomyelitis because it enhances the host's own immune system, and not because it kills the bacteria directly.[5]

There are many other reports of controlled HBOT studies, all emphasizing that HBOT is an excellent supplement to good surgical and antibiotic management. The overall success rate in various investigations using HBOT on osteomyelitis ranges from 60 percent to 85 percent, with a lower rate of recurrence.

HBOT has also proven its worth in human treatment. Dr. Jefferson C. Davis, a leading figure in the early days of hyperbaric medicine, studied two groups of patients— 98 in 1977 and 38 in 1986—at the Southwest Texas Methodist Hospital. These patients had refractory chronic osteomyelitis of the spine, extremities, pelvis, skull, and chest wall. Each had experienced a failure of surgical and antibiotic treatment. In over half of all these patients, the infections cleared up completely as a result of receiving HBOT. They remained cured long after a five-year follow-up study was completed.[6,7] It's significant to note that from mid-1991 to the end of 1993, 417 patients underwent a total of 11,371 treatments in the hyperbaric oxygen chamber at this same hospital. Without this therapy, many of them would have lost their limbs—and others, their lives.

In another study, 40 patients suffering from chronic osteomyelitis were treated with HBOT as an adjunct to surgery and antibiotics. The cure rate at the two-year follow-up examination was 85 percent.[8]

As we have already mentioned, osteomyelitis can develop in the jawbone after tooth extraction. HBOT has also proven its worth in these cases. In one published report, HBOT was used for intractable osteomyelitis in 3 dental patients, and the therapy proved highly successful.[9] Three years later, 3 other patients were treated in a different treatment facility for the same condition. All 3 patients were healed, but the time it took depended on the extent of the infection. One patient saw results in six months, another in thirteen months, and a third after two years of HBOT.[10]

A good three-part treatment plan for osteomyelitis includes the use of antibiotics, surgery to remove dead bone when necessary, and HBOT as a supporting, or adjunct, treatment. The hyperbaric oxygen should be given at 2.4 atmospheres absolute once a day, for a minimum of sixty treatments.

WHEN BONES BECOME INFLAMED: ASEPTIC BONE NECROSIS

Under certain circumstances, bones can become inflamed without being infected. Such an inflammation is called *aseptic bone necrosis* (ABN). This painful condition occurs most often among professional divers, but is also a growing problem among recreational divers. It is usually a complication of decompression sickness (see Chapter 1). Yet it can also occur as a complication of a number of other diseases, including diabetes, hepatitis, rheumatoid arthritis, and sickle cell anemia. In addition, it can result as a side effect of various therapeutic procedures, such as radiation therapy and steroid treatment.

Aseptic bone necrosis disease can also occur spontaneously in the general population,[11-16] especially among children ages eight to fourteen. Among these patients, it behaves in a manner similar to Osgood-Schlatter disease, a childhood disorder affecting the bone section where growth takes place. This disease is characterized by various abnormalities of the growing bone and causes several symptoms, including pain, swelling, and joint disturbances, depending on what bones are involved. Osgood-Schlatter has no known cause, and neither does spontaneous ABN.

ABN is essentially a blood-supply problem.[17] Blood flow within the bone can be disrupted by a number of conditions, including decompression sickness (see Chapter 1) and trauma.

The blood-vessel obstruction results in ischemia, or reduced blood supply. This reduction means that the bone doesn't get enough nutrients and oxygen, and that cellular wastes accumulate. This causes the degeneration seen in ABN.

If not properly treated, ABN often involves multiple joints and often results in permanent disability. A patient can conceivably develop ABN in one hip and then have it involve the other hip, the shoulders, and the knees. Widespread ABN requires a great deal of joint-replacement surgery, and causes an incalculable amount of expense, pain, and disability for the patient.

Since a reduction in blood flow and resultant lack of oxygen are at the heart of the problem, it stands to reason that putting more oxygen in the affected tissues will help halt further deterioration and promote healing. There is evidence that HBOT does indeed help patients with ABN. Dr. Neubauer and his colleagues treated a patient, a recreational diver, by giving him HBOT over an extended period of time. After thirty-eight sessions, the man's pain was relieved. However, his problems recurred, and he was treated with another, longer HBOT series. The patient eventually received a total of 108 HBOT sessions, and had lasting relief thereafter.

As a result, the Neubauer team concluded that any treatment of ABN definitely requires long-term HBOT.[18] Short-term HBOT, involving only an average of twenty sessions, docs relieve the pain and disability of patients with ABN. However, no lasting cure takes place.[19,20] This conclusion is supported by another study, in which a patient with ABN in the hip found long-term relief after 120 HBOT treatments.[21]

The best treatment for ABN consists of daily ninety-minute exposures at 2.2 to 2.8 atmospheres absolute (see "The Language of HBOT and of Research" on page 7). The course of the disease and its treatment should be monitored by periodic MRI and x-ray examinations (see "Peering Within the Body" on page 23).

WHEN BROKEN BONES WON'T HEAL: FRACTURE NONUNION

In most cases of bone fracture, the bone regenerates itself and heals the break. (See "Different Types of Fractures" on page 85.) In some cases, however, the bone fails to heal. That is called a *fracture nonunion*.

HBOT works to heal fracture nonunion by stimulating the production of collagen, a tough, fibrous material that fills in the space between the two broken ends of bone. Collagen production, in turn, stimulates the production of capillaries, the tiny blood vessels that connect arteries to veins. The more blood vessels there are in the area, the more oxygen and nutrients can be brought to the site of the break. This additional oxygen and nutrient supply reinvigorates the cells that break down old bone and form new bone, and stimulates the formation of calcium deposits within the newly formed bone.[22–24]

The extra blood vessels stimulated by HBOT help strengthen the dense, fibrous outer layer of bone, called the periosteum. With a good blood supply, HBOT nourishes this hard protective covering, which then renews the bone underneath.[25]

Animal studies have demonstrated HBOT's effectiveness in cases of fracture nonunion. Researchers have worked with rats, rabbits, and embryonic chicks, and have found that HBOT leads to greater cartilage production (cartilage is the material that separates bones from each other, such as in the knee) and increased bone formation.[26–28] HBOT also helps bone grafts—pieces of bone transplanted from one part of the patient's body to the other—to take hold. In 53 dogs that had undergone reconstructive leg grafts, high-pressure HBOT helped to improve bone regeneration when used early in the postoperative period.[29] In another animal study of 487 fractures in and around the joints, the researchers concluded that adding HBOT to conventional orthopedic methods shortened the process of bone regeneration and wound healing by ten to twelve days.[30]

HBOT has also been used with good results on at least one human patient with fracture nonunion. Dr. Neubauer and his colleague, Dr. J.R. Maxfield, Sr., treated a man with two broken bones in the lower leg that had not healed for thirty-three months (see Figure 8.1). Amputation had been recommended. Instead, the man received sixty one-hour HBOT sessions at 2.2 atmospheres absolute, over a period of thirty-eight days. The patient was periodically examined with x-rays. On the thirty-eighth day, pictures showed a healed fracture (see Figure 8.2). Follow-up sessions were given for two months afterwards to assure a complete healing process. With HBOT, the patient was able to return to work in less than four months. A final x-ray taken two-and-a-half years after the beginning of the HBOT series showed complete healing of the man's bone.[31]

In cases of fracture nonunion, HBOT should be given at 2.2 atmospheres absolute (see "The Language of HBOT and of Research" on page 7), in ninety-minute sessions for between forty-five and sixty days. Progress must be followed with sequential x-rays.

In this chapter, we've seen how HBOT can help heal several bone disorders that often occur as complications of accidents. In the next chapter, we'll study how HBOT can help control the complications that sometimes follow two forms of medical treatment: radiation therapy and skin surgery.

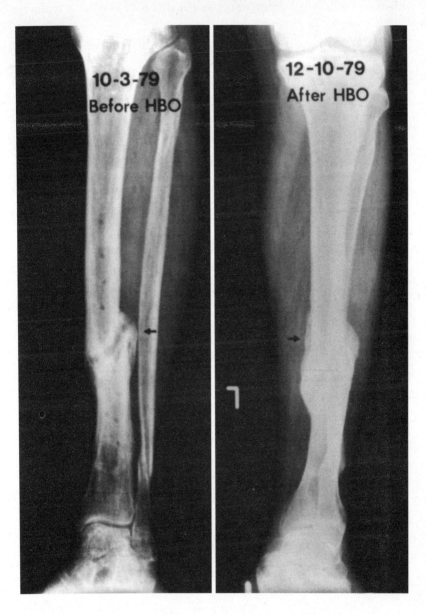

Figure 8.1.
Fracture Nonunion

Figure 8.2.
Same Fracture After HBOT

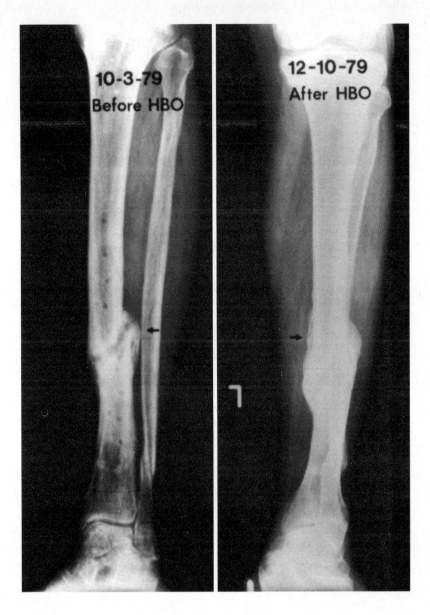

Figure 8.1.
Fracture Nonunion

Figure 8.2.
Same Fracture After HBOT

CHAPTER 9

Using HBOT to Treat Complications of Radiation Treatment and Skin Surgery

In Florida, 67-year-old Nellie D. receives radiation therapy for a cancer in her mouth. As a result, her jawbone is weakened, and spontaneously breaks. She has surgery to place a metal splint in her jaw. Unfortunately, the skin over the jaw has also been damaged, and Nellie is left with a hole in her skin, through which the splint is visible. An attempted skin graft fails. Another skin graft is attempted, but this time, Nellie receives twenty sessions of HBOT before the surgery and ten sessions afterwards. The graft is successful, and Nellie no longer needs to cover up an open wound.

Certain types of medical treatments and procedures can produce various types of complications. In some cases, HBOT can help patients recover from such complications more quickly than they could otherwise.

Each year, Americans undergo about 20 million radiation treatments, at an average of twenty-four treatments a patient. These people are subject to a number of side effects that HBOT can alleviate. Also, more than 1.5 million Americans undergo cosmetic surgery each year. HBOT may help these patients avoid complications, and can be extremely useful when problems do occur. (See Appendix A for information on contacting hyperbaric oxygen facilities.)

USING HBOT TO ALLEVIATE THE SIDE EFFECTS OF RADIATION TREATMENT

The body's cells are constantly renewing themselves. Radiation treatment damages cells by interfering with their ability to reproduce. If the cells cannot reproduce, they eventually die. That is why radiation treatment is used to treat cancer in the first place—cancer cells reproduce much more rapidly than normal cells do, and are thus more susceptible to radiation than normal cells are.

The idea of radiation treatment is to irradiate tumors with minimal damage to the surrounding normal tissue. However, it is almost impossible to direct radiation so precisely that none of the body's normal cells are affected. Radiation damage, called *radionecrosis*, may be the result. Radionecrosis can be easily induced by injury or surgery (even tooth extraction) after the patient has undergone radiation treatment.

Radiation damage tends to occur in four stages:[1]

- The *acute stage* occurs during the first six months of exposure to radiation. In this period, organs are damaged, but the damage is not noticeable.

- The *subacute stage* occurs during the second six months. As treatment continues, permanent tissue damage becomes evident.

- The *chronic stage* covers the second to fifth year after radiation exposure. At this point, residual tissue damage is apparent. There is deterioration of the capillaries, the tiny blood vessels that connect arteries to veins. This results in reduced blood and oxygen flow, and in the buildup of cell wastes. In turn, organ function is reduced and resistance to infection is lowered.

- The *late clinical stage* occurs following the fifth year after radiation exposure. This period is marked by premature aging and new, radiation-induced cancer growth.

Hyperbaricists are most concerned with localized radiation-induced damage. This damage generally appears during the subacute and chronic stages.

Until recently, there has been no satisfactory treatment of radiation damage. HBOT fills this long-standing need. Radiation damage causes hypoxia, or a lack of oxygen in the body's tissues. Hyperbaric oxygen helps fight this damage by increasing the amount of oxygen within the tissues, which aids in recovery. For example, extra oxygen stimulates the skin to form new collagen, the basic building material used in wound healing. New collagen, in turn, enhances the formation of new capillaries, supporting skin grafts and allowing small skin ulcers to heal over (see pages 103 and 104).

HBOT's usefulness in treating radiation damage was first reported in the medical literature in 1973, and has been documented in other reports since then.[2,3] In one important study written by Dr. George Hart and Dr. M.B. Strauss in the 1980s, 336 patients were treated with HBOT as an adjunct to surgery and other medical procedures following radiation treatment. Oxygen was given at 2.0 atmospheres absolute for two hours once a day in the case of outpatients, or 1.5 atmospheres absolute twice a day in the case of inpatients, for a total of 120 hours or less of HBOT. (See "The Language of HBOT and of Research" on page 7.) If healing was not adequate, the treatment was repeated after a three- to six-month rest period.[4] It is important to note that the researchers did not administer HBOT immediately following radiation because it might enhance the effects of the radiation if used too soon afterwards. Instead, the doctors started HBOT two months or more after each patient's last radiation treatment. The HBOT caused a marked reduction in the amount of disease among these patients when compared with what could normally be expected.

Radiation damages different tissues in different ways. There are two basic types of radiation damage: soft-tissue damage and bone damage. Let us see how HBOT can help treat each type.

HBOT and Soft-Tissue Damage

We will discuss the following kinds of soft-tissue radiation damage:

- Nervous-system damage

- Head and neck damage

- Genitourinary tract damage

- Miscellaneous soft-tissue damage

Radiation myelitis and *radiation encephalopathy* are two potential nervous-system complications of radiation treatment. Myelitis is an inflammatory disease that affects the entire spinal cord. This inflammation results in a loss of the cord's ability to transmit nerve impulses, much as if the cord had been severed. Myelitis following radiation treatment for throat cancer was reported in 1948 by Dr. G. Boden.[5] Encephalopathy is a disease that affects the functioning of the brain.

These complications develop when radiation damages capillaries in the spinal cord and brain. Blood clots form, which in turn reduces blood flow and causes a lack of oxygen in the tissues. By putting extra oxygen into the bloodstream, HBOT can overcome this lack. However, HBOT, if used too soon after radiation treatments are given, can aggravate the effects of radiation.[6,7] This means that HBOT has to be used very carefully, since adverse nervous-system effects may not appear for several months following the completion of radiation treatments.

Human patients have responded well to HBOT. One study looked at 23 patients who were given HBOT in the late stage of radiation-induced brain disease. The researchers examined blood-flow changes in the brains of these patients. Varying degrees of improvement was observed in all of the patients.[8]

Another study examined the cases of 10 patients with myelitis and 2 patients with encephalopathy. These patients received HBOT at 2.0 atmospheres absolute for ninety minutes per session, twice a day for two weeks. Three of the 10 myelitis patients had established neurological difficulties, and did not respond to treatment. Three others were treated with HBOT within one year after symptoms appeared. In these patients, the disease stopped progressing, and they showed slight improvement in their neurological problems. The remaining 4 myelitis patients had suffered symptoms for less than six months, and showed marked improvement after receiving HBOT. The 2 patients with encephalopathy were treated with vasodilators, drugs that help open up blood vessels, in addition to HBOT. They also showed marked improvement. As in other studies, the researchers conclude that HBOT is beneficial in treating these conditions but should not be given immediately following the radiation. They suggest that at least eight months should pass following the last radiation treatment.[9]

Radiation can not only damage the nervous system, but can also affect other soft tissues of the head and neck. For example, radionecrosis of the larynx (voice box) is a debilitating disease that results in pain, difficulty in swallowing, and respiratory obstruction. A laryngectomy, or removal of the larynx, is required in some cases. In a study by Dr. B.J. Ferguson, Dr. W.R. Hudson, and Dr. J.C. Farmer, 7 of 8 patients with advanced radionecrosis of the larynx treated with HBOT saw their symptoms sharply reduced. Only one patient required a laryngectomy.[10]

In another study, 48 patients underwent surgery after receiving radiation treatment to the head and neck. Their surgical wounds opened up because of radiation-induced damage to the tissues. These patients were given HBOT and all except one of the patients improved.[11]

Radiation treatment can also damage the genitourinary tract. Blood in the urine is the main symptom. It often takes the form of *cystitis*, or inflammation of the bladder. Secondary infection is almost always present.

Conventional treatment of this complication has included various types of drugs, but has not been effective to any degree. However, HBOT works well. For instance, Dr. D.J. Bakker and Dr. B.G. Rijkmans reported on 10 patients with radiation-induced cystitis who were treated with oxygen at 3.0 atmospheres absolute for ninety minutes a day, five sessions a week for an average of four weeks. Five patients saw their urinary bleeding stop after twelve HBOT sessions. In the other 5, bleeding was reduced, but did not stop. In these patients, residual tumors were found in the bladder. HBOT had reduced swelling in the surrounding tissue, which made the tumors easier to find. These tumors were then removed.[12]

In another study, 15 patients had radiation damage to the bladder. Eleven of these patients were relieved of bleeding and a constant desire to defecate (which indicates bowel damage) through a combination of HBOT and surgery.[13] And in a third study by Dr. J.B. Weiss and Dr. E.C. Neville, 8 patients who had been suffering from radiation-induced cystitis were treated with a series of two-hour HBOT sessions at 2.0 atmospheres absolute. They reported relief of symptoms, and this was confirmed by examination of their bladders, which showed significant reversal of tissue injury. Remissions took place in an average of twenty-four months, and only one patient failed to respond.[14]

Miscellaneous soft-tissue damage affects various locations in the body. Radiation that strikes a blood vessel can bring about swelling, degeneration, and death of the vessel lining, with resulting thickening of the vessel walls. The capillaries and the smallest arteries suffer the most damage, whereas the larger blood vessels may be spared. During the chronic third stage of radiation damage, the skin often atrophies, and ulcers are likely to develop after minor bumps and bruises. Skin incisions made through radiation-affected areas heal poorly. The gastrointestinal tract may also become inflamed.

Again, studies have shown that people with miscellaneous soft-tissue damage can be helped by HBOT. In one example, 8 patients were healed of radiation-induced skin damage when skin grafts were used following HBOT (see page 103).[15] In another, HBOT was used to treat 20 patients who had radiation damage of the soft tissues. In 16 of these patients, the injuries healed.[16]

In cases of soft-tissue damage, HBOT is generally used at 2.4 atmospheres absolute (see "The Language of HBOT and of Research" on page 7) in ninety-minute sessions. Between twenty and thirty sessions are usually given, depending on the patient's response. Soft-tissue damage can also cause problems when a patient who has received head and neck radiation needs to undergo dental work. In this type of case, the patient generally receives twenty HBOT sessions before dental treatment and ten sessions afterwards.

HBOT and Bone Damage

Radiation can also damage bone. Since bone is 1.6 times more dense than soft tissue, it absorbs a larger portion of a radiation dose than does soft tissue. High doses of radiation can damage the blood vessels passing between the membrane covering the bone and the surface of the bone itself, which leads to bone death. Radiation can also upset the balance between the destruction and construction of bone, which occurs constantly. This leads to brittleness and, finally, death of the bone, which appears between four months and three years following radiation. (For more information on HBOT and bone damage, see Chapter 8.) The usual sites of radiation-induced bone damage are:

- The lower jawbone, or mandible, generally following radiation treatment of soft tissue tumors of the head and neck.

- The ribs and the breastbone, or sternum, usually following radiation treatment of breast cancer.

- The spinal column, usually following radiation of spinal cord tumors.

The jawbone is often damaged by radiation treatment, for two reasons. First, it is denser than the other facial bones, which means that it absorbs more radiation than they do. Second, the jawbone has a limited blood supply compared with other facial bones. As a result, radiation damage of the jawbone is the most commonly reported form of bone damage. In one study, it happened in 235 of 378 patients, or 62.2 percent.[17] Damage to an irradiated jawbone may take a number of forms, including pathological fracture, in which the bone breaks under little or no stress. In some cases, x-rays do not show any abnormalities and even if abnormalities are present, they may not correlate with the severity of the patient's symptoms. Such symptoms can include pain, tooth loss, dry mouth, and gum sores.

In the past, infection was thought to play a role in radiation-induced jawbone damage. However, antibiotics have not been very effective in reversing this condition. In one study, only 8 percent of the patients who had surgery and took antibiotics achieved remission of their symptoms.[18] It is now generally believed that infection does not play an important role in this process.

In contrast to antibiotics, HBOT has proven its worth in the treatment of radiation-induced jawbone damage. Hart and Strauss reported on 206 patients who received HBOT as an adjunct treatment. Of these patients, 72 percent responded with excellent results, 10 percent with good results, and 15 percent with fair results. The remaining 3 percent did not respond.[19]

In 1985, one expert in the field, Dr. Robert Marx, and his colleagues conducted a study that involved cancer patients who were at a high risk for radiation-induced jawbone damage after tooth extraction. Some members of the group received only penicillin before and after tooth extraction. The others received no antibiotics, but did get HBOT at 2.4 atmospheres absolute in ninety-minute sessions a day for twenty days, half before extraction and the other half afterwards. The incidence of radiation damage was 29.9 percent in the antibiotic group and only 5.4 percent in the HBOT group.[20]

Radiation-induced damage to the chest wall is another fairly common complication of radiation treatment. It most commonly results from treatment for breast cancer, but can also occur after treatment for lung cancer or cancer of the mediastinum, the space in the chest between the two lung sacs. It usually produces soft tissue damage. However, large amounts of radiation may also weaken the ribs to the extent that coughing can cause a fracture.

In a study done by Dr. T. Kaufman, Dr. B. Hirshowitz, and Dr. I. Monies-Chass, 3 patients with radiation-induced damage of the chest wall were successfully treated with a combination of HBOT and surgery.[21] And in a 1986 study, researchers looked at 20 patients who received HBOT for this condition. All the patients made good recoveries.[22]

Another fairly common site of radiation-induced bone damage is the spinal column, which is made up of thirty-three vertebrae. These vertebrae are divided into four groupings—neck, chest, lower back, and tailbone—and the location of the damage depends on where the cancer under treatment is located. Such damage causes back pain. There may also be impairment to the spinal cord itself. In a 1986 study, 4 patients with radiation-induced vertebrae damage were given HBOT, and some damaged tissue was removed. All four patients recovered.[23]

Dr. Marx developed a three-stage treatment plan at the University of Miami:[24]

- In *Stage I,* treatment includes daily ninety-minute HBOT sessions at 2.4 atmospheres absolute for thirty days, and saline rinses for wounds. No bone is removed, and no antibiotics are given. If the patient improves, ten further sessions of HBOT are given. If there is no improvement, the patient is reclassified as Stage II. Patients with severe symptoms are immediately classified as Stage III.

- In *Stage II,* dead tissue is removed from the wound to determine the need for and possible extent of surgery.

Ten further HBOT sessions are given. If healing takes place, the patient is called a Stage II respondee. If the wound opens up or fails to heal, the patient is reclassified as Stage III.

- In *Stage III*, the patient receives thirty HBOT treatments, followed by surgery to remove dead bone and to stabilize the jaw. Ten more HBOT treatments are given, and the patient is advanced to Stage III-R for surgical reconstruction of the jaw. *Stage III-R* emphasizes early reconstructive surgery and rehabilitation. Ten sessions with HBOT are administered in the postoperative period and jaw fixation is maintained for eight weeks.

Dr. Marx and his colleagues treated 268 patients over a period of eight years using this plan. Good results were achieved in all cases: 38 Stage I patients (14 percent), 48 Stage II patients (18 percent), and 182 Stage III patients (68 percent).

PREVENTING THE COMPLICATIONS OF SKIN SURGERY WITH HBOT

Skin surgery is performed for a variety of reasons, from the removal of skin cancers to the repair of disfigurements. (The latter category includes disfigurements that result from burns—see Chapter 7.) However, much skin surgery falls into the category of cosmetic surgery, or surgery to improve one's appearance. Such surgery is becoming more and more popular, especially among career-minded professionals—there has been a 230 percent surge in cosmetic operations in the United States since 1981.

One reason cosmetic surgery has become more popular is that new surgical techniques have made such surgery more effective and less risky. What's more, the use of HBOT can help assure that skin grafts take hold and scars don't reveal themselves. Healing takes place three times faster than before HBOT became available to plastic surgeons. In this section, we will look at how HBOT can help patients undergoing three types of skin procedures: skin grafts, skin ulcer treatment, and laser surgery for port wine stains.

Skin surgery often requires the use of skin grafts, in which skin is taken from one part of the patient's body and used to cover a break in the skin on another part. There are several types of skin grafts. They include *full-thickness grafts*, in which all of the skin layers are used, and *split-thickness grafts*, in which only the top layers and several of the deeper layers are used. There are also *pedicle grafts*, in which part of the skin remains attached to the donor site. This allows the old blood supply to remain intact while a new blood supply develops.

One problem that has always vexed plastic surgeons is what to do when skin grafts do not survive, or "take." A freshly applied split-thickness graft receives no oxygen until tiny blood vessels called capillaries can penetrate into it. Such capillary ingrowth normally takes place over a two- to three-day period. If this does not happen, it's not likely that the graft will survive. HBOT tends to improve the chances that a graft will take, both by supplying oxygen directly to the graft and by encouraging quick capillary growth.

Lack of oxygen tends to be less of a problem with full-thickness and pedicle grafts, since these grafts have their own supply of capillaries. Even so, it still takes time for good blood flow to become established through these types of grafts. Therefore, full-thickness and pedicle grafts also respond to HBOT. In the case of a pedicle graft, it is important that HBOT be employed before what little circulation that is present develops blood clots.[25]

In many instances, HBOT is used only after a skin graft starts to fail. While HBOT can help save failing grafts, it can be even more effective when used before surgery to keep grafts from failing in the first place.

HBOT's effectiveness in aiding skin graft survival is supported by research. One of the first studies in this area was done in 1961, by pioneering reconstruction surgeon

Dr. Isadore Boerema. The grafts created by Dr. Boerema and his colleagues were in acute danger of being lost until HBOT was administered, after which all of them survived with good results.[26]

One researcher, Dr. J. David Perrins, did several studies in the 1960s. In 1966, Dr. Perrins studied the use of HBOT in a hospital unit where the usual failure rate for cosmetic surgery was 10 percent. With HBOT, the failure rate was reduced to 4.5 percent. Dr. Perrins recommended starting HBOT when there was any doubt as to the viability of the graft.[27] The next year, Dr. Perrins published results of a study that showed a higher proportion of successful complete skin grafts among patients who received HBOT (64 percent) compared with patients who did not (17 percent).[28] And in 1970, Dr. Perrins wrote about a controlled, single-blind study among patients who were receiving split-skin grafts. (See "The Language of HBOT and of Research" on page 7.) Directly after surgery, the patients were divided into two groups. One group was treated conventionally, and did not receive HBOT. The other received 100 percent oxygen at 2.0 atmospheres absolute for two hours, twice a day for three days. The latter group had the better results. Among these patients, an average of 92 percent of the surface area of the graft survived, compared with only 63 percent among the patients who did not receive HBOT.[29] These results have been supported by other studies.[30,31]

Before surgery, ten to forty HBOT sessions—2.0 atmospheres absolute for two hours each—can help keep a graft from failing. The patient can also be given HBOT two times a day for three days after surgery. The pressure is raised until the patient's skin graft is pink, and the elevated pressure is held at that level for sixty to ninety minutes.

HBOT can also help speed the healing of skin ulcers, especially chronic ulcers caused by a lack of oxygen. Such ulcers are often related to either blood-vessel disease (see

Chapter 11) or diabetes. It has been known since 1969 that even moderately elevated levels of oxygen may be effective in such situations.[32-35] HBOT not only helps the body develop new circulation in the wound area, as it does in skin grafts, but also inhibits or kills surface bacteria on the ulcers. (See Chapter 6 for information on how HBOT helps fight infections.) This therapy can also be used to prepare large or persistent ulcers for skin grafts.

For skin ulcers, a pressure between 2.0 and 2.4 atmospheres absolute is used for between ninety minutes and two hours a session. Treatment is given once or twice a day until the ulcer is either healed or ready for grafting. Diabetic ulcers can be very persistent, however, and can require eighty or more treatments. Some diabetic ulcer patients need 300 HBOT sessions before total healing takes place. It is important to remember that each patient is different.

HBOT is also used along with laser surgery to remove birthmarks known as port wine stains. In newborns, such stains are flat with a pink or red coloration. The stains tend to darken and take on a raised or lumpy appearance throughout adolescence and adulthood. These birthmarks can lead to soft-tissue deformities and vascular tumors. Because they are unsightly, port wine stains may lead to psychological problems, especially if they appear on the face or hands.

Modern laser surgery destroys the enlarged and excess blood vessels of the port wine stain, while leaving surrounding normal tissue unaffected. The risk of scarring, formerly between 50 to 60 percent with older types of laser equipment, is now less than 2 percent. That small risk can be lowered even more if HBOT is used after surgery. Directly following the laser operation, and each day thereafter for at least three days, the patient is given HBOT at 2.0 atmospheres absolute for one hour. Laser treatment and HBOT can also be used together for other blood-vessel abnormalities, including benign tumors and broken veins.

In this chapter, we've seen how HBOT can help patients either avoid or recover from complications caused by radiation treatment and skin surgery. In the next chapter, we'll discuss how HBOT can be used to help patients recover from poisoning.

CHAPTER 10

Using HBOT to Treat Poisoning

A firefighter—he could be from anywhere—is brought to a hospital suffering from smoke inhalation. He shows signs of being poisoned by carbon monoxide, a toxic gas present in smoke. He is drowsy and confused, and his breathing is labored. SPECT scans of his brain show damage caused by a lack of oxygen. Under ideal conditions, he receives twenty-five or more HBOT treatments over the course of a couple of weeks. All the while, his brain scans are rechecked. When his scans are normal, and only then, does the firefighter go back on active duty.

One of HBOT's most useful applications is as an antidote for certain types of poisoning. Each year, Americans are rushed to emergency rooms more than 800,000 times after encounters with various poisons, from children who ingest household chemicals to adults who are overcome by carbon monoxide fumes. HBOT helps reverse the poisonous effects of a number of different toxic substances.

In this chapter, we'll first see how HBOT is used to treat carbon monoxide poisoning, the most common form of poisoning. We'll then see how HBOT assists people poisoned by other substances. (See Appendix A for information on contacting hyperbaric oxygen facilities.)

CARBON MONOXIDE AND HBOT

Carbon monoxide—a colorless, odorless gas—is the most common cause of death by poisoning. Thousands of Americans die of carbon monoxide poisoning every year, and more than 10,000 people miss at least one day of work because of exposure to carbon monoxide. The gas is produced by motor vehicles, defective gas appliances, and factories. It is also produced during fires and mining accidents, and by propane-powered equipment. Also, methylene chloride, the active ingredient in paint thinner, is converted to carbon monoxide by enzymes in the liver.

The severity of the symptoms produced by carbon monoxide poisoning depends on the concentration of gas and the length of exposure. Low concentrations bring on the symptoms of mild poisoning: headache, dizziness, confusion, irritability, and lack of concentration. Moderate concentrations produce drowsiness and sight impairment. High concentrations produce severe symptoms, including seizures and coma, and can cause death. Other symptoms include marked breathing difficulties and, rarely, a cherry-pink color to the skin.

Some people are subject to chronic, low-level carbon monoxide poisoning. These include smokers (see "Cigarettes and Carbon Monoxide" on page 110) and toll collectors breathing car exhaust at highways, bridges, and tunnels. Because the damage done by chronic carbon monoxide poisoning is cumulative, it can impair mental function. Its late effects include dementia and psychiatric disturbances, physical movement disorders, and extreme drowsiness. Symptoms can recur weeks or months after an acute episode of carbon monoxide poisoning.

Carbon monoxide poisoning has been called "the great imitator." It is frequently misdiagnosed because it mimics many other conditions. As a result, patients may return to the very environments that brought on their symptoms in the first place.

Carbon monoxide produces its poisonous effects by displacing and substituting for oxygen. Normally, red blood cells transport oxygen throughout the body. These cells carry a substance called *hemoglobin*, which binds to oxygen in the lungs and releases that oxygen to the body's tissues. When carbon monoxide is inhaled, it attaches to hemoglobin with a tie that is 240 times greater than oxygen's tie to hemoglobin. Thus, the red blood cell that picks up carbon monoxide cannot carry any oxygen. When enough red blood cells take on carbon monoxide, the amount of oxygen in the bloodstream drops, and the body's tissues become starved for oxygen.[1] This effect is cumulative: a concentration of only 0.1 percent carbon monoxide will cause serious symptoms if inhaled for one hour.

Without oxygen, cells cannot produce energy. Without energy, cell function decreases, and the cells begin to poison themselves with their own waste. Carbon monoxide also penetrates into the brain cells themselves. As elsewhere in the body, a lack of oxygen often leads to swelling, and in the brain, this swelling causes even more brain tissue to be destroyed. Thus, the brain is particularly affected by carbon monoxide.[2] This accounts for the drowsiness and mental effects (whether immediate or delayed) seen in carbon monoxide poisoning.[3-8]

Another organ that is particularly affected by carbon monoxide poisoning is the heart, which, like the brain, needs a lot of oxygen. The heart is especially vulnerable to the toxic effects of carbon monoxide because the gas binds to the heart muscle three times more strongly than it binds to other muscles in the body. People with heart disease already have hearts that are not working at full capacity, and are therefore more susceptible to carbon monoxide poisoning.

HBOT is well established as a highly effective treatment for carbon monoxide poisoning. It puts so much extra oxygen into the bloodstream that the body's hemoglobin is forced to bind with oxygen instead of carbon monoxide. Some of the extra oxygen dissolves in the blood plasma, which usually doesn't carry oxygen. This puts even more

Cigarettes and Carbon Monoxide

There are many well-documented hazards associated with smoking, such as higher risks for both lung and bladder cancer. There are also smoking-related hazards that you may not have heard about. One of those hidden hazards is low-level carbon monoxide poisoning.

As in the case of smoke inhalation, the carbon monoxide produced by smoking is a product of combustion, since a cigarette is basically a low-level fire. There are between 14 and 23 milligrams of carbon monoxide in each unfiltered cigarette. This carbon monoxide affects not only the smoker, but also those who breathe that person's smoke.

The carbon monoxide from cigarettes, as from any other source, ties up the bloodstream's oxygen-carrying hemoglobin, rendering it unable to carry oxygen. The body does produce some carbon monoxide as a normal waste product, so an average nonsmoker has between 0.5 and 1.5 percent of his or her hemoglobin tied up by carbon monoxide. But among smokers, according to one study, that number goes up to 4.7 percent.*

The best way to avoid this source of carbon monoxide poisoning is, of course, not to start smoking, or to quit if you have started. A wide variety of smoking cessation aids is available, from nicotine patches and gums, to behavior-modification programs and books such as *No If's, And's, or Butts*, to hypnosis and biofeedback. It is also wise to spend most of your time in a smoke-free environment. The addiction to tobacco can be a difficult addiction to break, but your lungs—and your hemoglobin—will thank you.

----

*Source: *Reducing the Health Consequences of Smoking*, U.S. Department of Health and Human Services, 1989, p. 96.

oxygen into the body's tissues. HBOT reduces swelling and can counteract the breakdown of brain cells that contributes to the neurological symptoms associated with carbon monoxide poisoning.

The use of HBOT can reduce carbon monoxide's half-life, or the length of time it takes for half of the poison to leave the body. The half-life of carbon monoxide in the bloodstream is 5.3 hours when breathing regular air at sea level. The use of HBOT at 3.0 atmospheres absolute reduces the half-life to twenty-three minutes.

Evidence of HBOT's effectiveness in counteracting carbon monoxide was first discovered in 1895. In that year, a famous Scottish physiologist, Dr. John Scott Haldane, put a mouse in a jar containing 2.0 atmospheres absolute of oxygen and 1.0 atmospheres absolute of carbon monoxide. The mouse showed no noticeable symptoms of poisoning (see "The Language of HBOT and of Research" on page 7).[9] In 1942, pioneering hyperbaricist Dr. Edgar End and his colleague, Dr. C.W. Long, were the first to show that high-pressure oxygen was more effective than normal-pressure oxygen in treating carbon monoxide poisoning.[10] A number of subsequent animal studies clearly demonstrated that hyperbaric oxygen could drive carbon monoxide out of its bonds with hemoglobin.[11,12]

Human beings affected by carbon monoxide poisoning were first treated with HBOT in 1960. The first two patients recovered completely.[13] As time went on, doctors learned that HBOT is useful as a life-saving measure even when there is a delay between gas exposure and treatment.[14]

In 1979, Dr. Neubauer treated a patient who had been in a coma for eleven days as the result of carbon monoxide poisoning. On the twelfth day, the patient began receiving HBOT. The patient had brain swelling and grossly abnormal brain waves. The man awoke during the first HBOT session. After the twenty-third session, he was able to walk without assistance and his mental symptoms improved. Eventually, he was able to return to a normal routine with only minimal aftereffects.[15] A number of other researchers went on to confirm Dr. Neubauer's experience.[16–20]

Some groups of people face a greater risk of carbon monoxide poisoning than others. While many people are exposed to low levels of carbon monoxide, firefighters are often exposed to high levels of the poisonous gas. Children and pregnant women are more susceptible to the effects of carbon monoxide. So are the elderly. All of these people can be helped by HBOT.

Flames and falls aren't the only dangers a firefighter faces. The smoke from a burning building contains many toxic substances, including cyanide (see page 115) and carbon monoxide. Smoke inhalation can be a life-threatening condition.[21]

Proper treatment of smoke inhalation should include the use of HBOT, as in the hypothetical case study at the beginning of this chapter. However, firefighters who are overcome by smoke are usually just given normal-pressure oxygen at the scene of the fire. Lab tests administered to such patients show only how much carbon monoxide is in the blood, and not how much is actually within the body's tissues. If the blood test shows a normal reading, frequently no further treatment is given. As a result, a certain percentage of these firefighters continue to have ongoing heart and brain problems from smoke inhalation. It is often said of these unfortunate victims that they "ate too much smoke."

Dr. Neubauer strongly believes that smoke-inhalation patients should be given HBOT in cases of severe exposure to carbon monoxide. The use of HBOT would help these patients avoid the residual brain damage caused by carbon monoxide poisoning. This is especially true if treatment is continued until a patient's SPECT scans become normal (see Chapter 2), which may take up to three or four weeks after the initial injury.[22] A 1989 report by Dr. S.R. Thom showed no residual damage among 500 patients treated with HBOT. In contrast, the incidence of brain damage was 12 percent in those treated with only normal-pressure oxygen.[23]

A 1989 report pointed out that carbon monoxide accounts for more than 50 percent of the approximately 12,000 fire-associated deaths that occur each year. HBOT can reduce that number.[24]

Children are more susceptible than adults to carbon monoxide poisoning. They are at a greater risk of suffering brain damage as a result of carbon monoxide exposure.[25,26] Children living in homes where the parents smoke heavily are predisposed to such problems (see page 110). Even without any history of exposure to high concentrations of carbon monoxide, the steady and intrusive quality of chronic exposure does subtle damage to the brain's tissues. Dr. Neubauer believes that this toxic exposure may be a source of the antisocial behavior exhibited by some children when they reach adolescence. If the problem is recognized, HBOT can help these children recover their mental capacities without side effects.[27]

A pregnant woman is especially prone to the effects of carbon monoxide because the fetus, which absorbs carbon monoxide through the placenta, eliminates the gas slowly. The use of HBOT is the best way to ensure that a pregnant patient receives this extra oxygen. At one time, doctors thought that HBOT might harm the fetus, but this has been definitively disproved. For example, in 1989, a 17-year-old pregnant woman suffering from carbon monoxide poisoning was rushed to a nearby hyperbaric chamber, where she was treated with HBOT for ninety minutes. The treatment saved the young woman's life, along with the life of her 37-week-old fetus. The patient recovered and produced a healthy baby at full term with a normal delivery. If the mother had not received HBOT, considerable brain damage might have resulted for both her and the baby, and the baby might not have survived at all.[28]

A pregnant patient should receive HBOT under the following conditions:

- She has a history of exposure with severe symptoms

- There are signs of fetal distress, such as an overly rapid heartbeat or other heartbeat irregularities

- There are continuing problems twelve hours after the initial HBOT treatment

Most hyperbaricists have concluded that HBOT is a useful treatment for carbon monoxide poisoning and smoke inhalation. The authors of one study advise that HBOT be used in the initial treatment of all patients with carbon monoxide poisoning regardless of its severity.[29] We've already seen what conditions would indicate the use of HBOT in the treatment of pregnant women. For other patients, it should be used under the following circumstances:

- When a patient has a history of becoming unconscious after exposure to smoke or carbon monoxide

- When tests show damage to bodily tissues or carbon monoxide levels above 15 percent

- If the SPECT scan is abnormal, or if the CAT scan or MRI shows brain swelling (see "Peering Within the Body" on page 23)

The first treatment, which should be given after exposure, should be at 3.0 atmospheres absolute (see "The Language of HBOT and of Science" on page 7) for one hour. The second treatment should be at 2.5 atmospheres absolute for one hour, and should be given within four to six hours of the first treatment if the patient is comatose or in a stupor. The third treatment should be at 2.0 atmospheres absolute, followed by ten treatments at 1.5 atmospheres absolute. The total number of treatments varies with each patient.

Many doctors believe that one session of HBOT is all that is needed in cases of carbon monoxide poisoning. However, one session does not do enough to protect the brain from the damage that can be caused by exposure to this noxious gas. In some cases, the patient may require up to sixty treatments. Unfortunately, the use of multiple treatments is not standard practice in the United States—as it is in mainland China, for instance—and many patients are left with permanent brain damage as a result. (For more information on brain damage, see Chapter 3.)

OTHER POISONS AND HBOT

While carbon monoxide is the most common poisoning agent, thousands of people are poisoned each year by many other substances. HBOT can counteract poisoning by the following agents:

- Cyanide
- Hydrogen sulfide
- Carbon tetrachloride

HBOT can also be used to counteract a condition called methemoglobinemia, in which the blood's ability to carry oxygen is reduced upon exposure to various substances.

Cyanide is one of the most rapidly acting lethal poisons known. Inhalation of minimal amounts of cyanide causes instantaneous death. A swallowed dose can cause death in one hour. A nonfatal dose causes vomiting, diarrhea, confusion, dizziness, headache, weakness, breathing difficulties, convulsions, and coma.

Most cases of cyanide poisoning happen as the result of suicide attempts. However, it can occur after industrial accidents, particularly in the electroplating industry, or during fumigation for pest control. In addition, it can be caused by a drug called sodium nitroprusside, prescribed for certain circulatory problems, or by smoke inhalation, since most plastics give off cyanide when burned. Autopsies of smoke inhalation victims frequently show toxic levels of cyanide.

In cyanide poisoning, the patient essentially suffocates because the body cannot use oxygen. HBOT works well with the standard cyanide antidote, which uses amyl nitrate and sodium nitrate, followed by sodium thiosulfate. Case studies (see "The Language of HBOT and of Research" on page 7) have shown HBOT to be an effective treatment for cyanide poisoning.[30,31]

Hydrogen sulfide is a highly toxic gas that is readily recognized by its characteristic "rotten eggs" odor. In high concentrations, it can cause death. At lower concentrations, it can irritate the eyes, throat, and lungs. Hydrogen sulfide can also cause headache, weakness, convulsions, a feeble pulse, and a fall in both body temperature and blood pressure. Chronic low-level exposure can bring on headache, nausea, confusion, insomnia, dry mouth, tearing, abdominal cramps, and throat and chest irritation.

Hydrogen sulfide has a number of industrial applications, including use as a bleaching agent. Most poisoning cases result from industrial exposure.

Like carbon monoxide, hydrogen sulfide ties up the hemoglobin in the body's oxygen-carrying red blood cells, which reduces the amount of oxygen that reaches the tissues. This loss of oxygen produces swelling of the brain, which can cause brain damage.

HBOT counteracts hydrogen sulfide by flooding the body with oxygen, therefore overcoming the oxygen depletion in the body's tissues, especially within the brain. Animal studies have proven that this use of hyperbaric oxygen is much more effective than the administration of normal-pressure oxygen. These studies have also shown that HBOT works best when combined with the antidote of amyl nitrate and sodium nitrate.[32] This combination has proven itself useful in treating human patients.[33-35]

Carbon tetrachloride (carbon tet) is a colorless, dense liquid that gives off poisonous fumes. When inhaled, it produces shallow breathing, clammy skin, low blood pressure, and a slow pulse. When swallowed, it causes headache, drowsiness, confusion, abdominal pain, thick speech, and a slow pulse. A patient may show very few symptoms until the liver and kidneys are damaged, at which point the person's chances of recovery are minimal.

Carbon tet is used in the dry-cleaning industry, and people who work in that industry are the ones who are most commonly poisoned. Carbon tet poisoning was more common among the general public before its sale as a home cleaning agent was banned.

Like other poisons, carbon tet causes a shortage of oxygen in the body's tissues. It also causes liver damage by producing substances known as free radicals, which bind to the liver's cells and render the cells unable to carry out their normal functions. In some cases, it can bring on complete liver failure. Carbon tet also has a toxic effect on the kidneys.

HBOT can counteract carbon tet by reducing liver damage, especially if given in combination with such free-radical neutralizers as the antioxidants selenium and vitamins C and E. Animal studies have shown that HBOT improves the survival rate, especially if used within an hour after exposure, and that survivors have less liver damage.[36,37]

A number of human patients have been successfully treated with HBOT.[38-40] In one case, treatment began twenty-four hours after the patient swallowed 150 milliliters—about 5 ounces—of carbon tetrachloride. HBOT was begun when severe liver damage was already present and the patient was near death. As a result of treatment with HBOT, the patient recovered. Amazingly, a biopsy of the liver taken on the twelfth day following the poisoning showed only minimal remaining liver damage.[41]

Many chemicals can produce *methemoglobinemia*, a condition in which red blood cells cannot carry their normal amount of oxygen because hemoglobin, the oxygen-bearing chemical they contain, is damaged. This condition degrades the ability of the body's tissues to get all the oxygen they need. Chemicals that can produce methemoglobinemia include nitrites and nitrates, used as preservatives in food and medicines; potassium chloride, used in fertilizer; potassium permanganate, used in dyes and deodorizers; drugs such as phenacetin, nitroglycerine, and local anesthetics; and aniline dyes.

Methemoglobinemia usually produces no symptoms, but is associated with collapse, coma, and death when it affects more than 65 percent of the blood's hemoglobin. While such deaths are rare, nonfatal levels of methemoglobinemia can cause people to function at less than full capacity.

HBOT is a proven treatment for methemoglobinemia, along with the antidote methylene blue. It has even been used for patients in drug-induced coma with blood levels of methemoglobin greater than 65 percent. Doctors are able to reduce methemoglobin levels in these patients by 6 percent an hour through the use of HBOT at 2.2 atmospheres absolute. The patients recover.[42-44]

All of the poisonings listed on page 115 can be counteracted with one-hour HBOT sessions, at 2.2 atmospheres absolute (see "The Language of HBOT and of Science" on page 7), every eight to twelve hours until the maximum benefit has occurred. Benefits can be determined by clinical examination of the patient, or by blood tests, SPECT scans, and EEGs. As many as thirty treatments may be required in some cases.

In this chapter, we've seen how HBOT can help patients who have been poisoned by a number of substances. As in the case of the other diseases and conditions we've discussed so far, hyperbaric oxygen's ability to aid poisoning victims lies in its ability to put more oxygen into all the body's fluids, including the blood. In the next chapter, we'll study how HBOT can be used to treat circulatory-system disease.

CHAPTER 11

Using HBOT to Treat Circulatory Problems

In Florida, 54-year-old Jewel C. has Raynaud's disease, which causes spasms in the arteries. She develops an extremely painful skin ulcer on her right index finger. After a period of wound care and medication to dilate the blood vessels, it is obvious that the ulcer is beginning to spread. Jewel's surgeon, concerned that she may lose her finger, refers her to a hyperbaric facility. In less than forty treatments, the ulcer is completely closed and the pain is relieved. The HBOT also relieves symptoms in Jewel's other fingers that are related to Raynaud's disease.

The heart and the major blood vessels, such as the aorta, make up only half of the circulatory system. The other half is made up of thousands of blood vessels throughout the body. When disease occurs in these blood vessels, it is called *peripheral vascular disease* (PVD). PVD may be a sign of a serious underlying condition, such as diabetes or heart disease. PVD can also have serious consequences, such as limb loss.[1] In the United States, according to the Department of Labor, PVD is responsible for more than 6 million person-days a year of lost work time.[2]

In this chapter, we'll first look at what causes circulatory problems, and then at how HBOT can be used to treat these problems. (See Appendix A for information on contacting hyperbaric oxygen facilities.)

WHAT CAUSES CIRCULATORY PROBLEMS?

The most common reason for circulatory problems is PVD, which is actually a group of diseases and conditions compromising blood flow to the extremities. PVD affects significant numbers of people. Among the industrialized nations, peripheral vascular diseases occur in 1.5 percent of those under forty years of age and in 5 percent of those over fifty years of age. In Germany, the number of hospitalization days for PVD is equal to the hospitalization days for cardiovascular diseases such as heart attack.[3]

The most notable symptom of PVD is limb pain. *Intermittent claudication* is pain in the calf or calves that is brought on by walking and relieved by rest. The more extensive the PVD, the shorter the distance a patient can walk before the pain starts. In severe cases of PVD, the pain may occur even when a patient is resting. Other signs of PVD include absent or weak pulse in the affected area, cold skin that is either pale or reddish blue, and, in extreme cases, skin ulcers or gangrene.

PVD includes a number of different conditions, including:

- *Arteriosclerosis obliterans.* In this condition, the patient has atherosclerosis (the accumulation of fatty plaques on the artery walls) in the extremities. Major risk factors for atherosclerosis include high blood pressure, high cholesterol, smoking, diabetes, obesity, and genetics.

- *Buerger's disease.* In this condition, also called thromboangiitis obliterans, arteries in the leg and foot become clotted and inflamed. Superficial veins are also affected. It mostly occurs in heavy smokers between the ages of twenty and forty. The symptoms include burning, numbness, and tingling.

- *Embolic or thrombotic occlusion.* In this condition, a small piece of fat or a blood clot becomes stuck in a blood vessel. This blocks the flow of blood to the affected limb. Often, the heart is the source of the clot.

- *Traumatic arterial occlusion.* In this condition, trauma to an artery interferes with blood flow to the affected limb. (For more information on trauma, see Chapter 5.)

- *Raynaud's disease.* In this condition, spasms occur in the arteries in the extremities, especially the fingers, toes, ears, and nose. It can be brought on by emotional upsets or exposure to cold. The skin turns pale, with a bluish tinge, and then turns red. There is numbness, tingling, and, often, pain. These problems are all caused by the reduction of blood flow in the affected limb.

- *Miscellaneous arterial diseases.* These conditions include blood-vessel damage caused by abuse of injectable drugs such as heroin, and by various forms of blood-vessel inflammation, including those related to allergies and to diseases such as lupus and other autoimmune conditions.

People with PVD are at a high risk for serious health problems, such as stroke and heart disease. That's because atherosclerosis occurs throughout the body, and not in any one body part. Thus, PVD of the lower limbs is recognized as a sign of cardiovascular disease.

The connection between PVD and life-threatening illness is borne out by research. Study results indicate that 50 percent of people with atherosclerosis show signs of it in many blood vessels throughout the body.[4] Someone who has PVD is likely to have atherosclerosis in the heart or aorta approximately 57 percent of the time, and in the blood vessels of the brain about 25 percent of the time.[5-9] Among patients with PVD resulting from atherosclerosis, the causes of death include severe coronary disease or heart attack (60 percent) and stroke (16 percent).[10,11] People with intermittent claudication run a higher risk of death than those without this condition.[12-15]

HOW HBOT EASES CIRCULATORY PROBLEMS

Conventional treatment of PVD has mostly consisted of dietary modification, exercise therapy (see page 124), and various types of surgery:

- *Angioplasty.* In this operation, a tube is placed into the affected vessel. The blockage is then either flattened by a tiny balloon, or destroyed by either a laser or by radio waves. The results are sometimes good in the short term, although improvements seldom hold over the long term.[16]

- *Endarterectomy.* In this operation, the blockage is removed from the blood vessel. It is usually done when the vessel is almost entirely blocked. This procedure does not work well when small vessels are involved.

- *Vein bypass or replacement.* In a bypass operation, blood flow is shunted around the affected section of the blood vessel. In a replacement operation, the affected section is entirely replaced. The shunt or replacement is either a synthetic vein or a vein taken from elsewhere in the patient's body. Like the endarterectomy, this operation does not work well on small vessels, although newer surgical techniques are being developed to overcome this limitation.

- *Sympathectomy.* In this operation, a nerve, usually in the upper thigh, is cut. This can cause tightened blood vessels to relax. It is an older procedure that is not often used anymore. However, it occasionally produces good results.

Sometimes, a strawlike tube called a stent is used to continue circulation through a blocked area. Drug treatment for PVD is also available. However, vasodilators—drugs that dilate blood vessels—have proven to be ineffective because they affect only normal vessels, and not vessels that have become constricted. One drug that does work is Trental (pentoxifylline), which changes the shape of the red blood cells so that they can slide more easily through narrowed blood vessels.

How can HBOT help treat PVD? As we've seen, PVD results in an inadequate flow of blood to the affected tissues, a condition known as ischemia. Usually, ischemia is caused by constriction or blockage of the blood vessels supplying the tissues, such as the constriction that results when a blood vessel is narrowed by atherosclerosis. When ischemia occurs, there is a reduction in the amount of oxygen that reaches the tissues. This reduction in tissue oxygen, which is called hypoxia, leads to swelling and, thus, further hypoxia.

HBOT helps patients with PVD in several ways.[17] The use of hyperbaric oxygen leads to the development of new capillaries, tiny blood vessels linking arteries and veins. This allows a greater amount of oxygen to be delivered to the affected tissues, which, in turn, results in more oxygen being absorbed by the tissues. Hypoxia is relieved and swelling decreases. Also, HBOT forces oxygen into the blood plasma and the lymph, which normally do not carry oxygen. This dissolved oxygen is more readily used by the body than the oxygen that is normally carried by the red blood cells.[18,19] That's because oxygen carried in fluid is immediately available to the body's cells, while oxygen in red blood cells requires the use of energy to make it available.

As a result of the additional oxygen, the tissues function more normally. The effects of HBOT can readily be seen in the way the patient's skin and nail beds steadily turn pink or red in color.[20] HBOT also improves the blood's chemical properties,[21-24] and appears to reduce the blood's tendency to clump.

Relief from hypoxia can help, in turn, relieve the pain often experienced by PVD patients. HBOT also acts to relieve pain by reducing the swelling that generally accompanies hypoxia, and by making it easier for the affected tissues to rid themselves of irritating cell wastes.

In addition to reducing hypoxia and pain, HBOT can also help reduce the incidence and extent of gangrene. This may save the affected limb from amputation. In cases where amputation is unavoidable, the use of HBOT can make the line of demarcation between living and dead tissues more obvious, thus allowing the surgeon to save as much tissue as possible. HBOT can also promote the healing of skin ulcers caused by reduced blood flow (see Chapter 9).

In the 1960s and into the 1970s, doctors disagreed about HBOT's ability to help PVD patients. That's because some early experiments did not show that HBOT helped improve the delivery of oxygen to the tissues.[25,26] However, other studies found that HBOT does improve oxygen delivery in diseased, oxygen-starved limbs.[27-31]

Even before the issue was fully settled in the laboratory, doctors were using HBOT to help patients. In 1962, Dr. C.F.W. Illingworth found that HBOT could help save limbs in patients with severe arterial injuries. He also noticed that HBOT could help relieve pain and heal skin ulcers in patients with PVD.[32] Other studies noted that HBOT helped reduce the amount of gangrenous tissue that had to be amputated.

In the 1980s and into the 1990s, additional doctors found HBOT to be useful in treating PVD, especially when used with other treatment methods. In France, Dr. P. Fredenucci worked with 2,021 patients between 1966 and 1983, and found that proper blood flow to underoxygenated parts of the body was revived in 40 percent of the patients treated with HBOT.[33] Other studies found that HBOT healed skin ulcers.[34-39]

One of the most useful roles HBOT has in PVD treatment is as an adjunct to exercise therapy. Dr. K.K. Jain did a pilot study in Germany involving four men, ranging in age from forty-nine to seventy, who had intermittent claudication. All four had been treated medically for PVD, although none had undergone surgery. For two years, they walked on a treadmill inside a hyperbaric oxygen chamber. The pressure used was 1.5 atmospheres absolute (see "The Language of HBOT and of Research" on page 7) in sessions lasting forty-five minutes. Sessions in plain air and 100 percent oxygen, both at normal pressures, were used as controls. Two of the patients were treated daily, while the other two were treated weekly.

The authors found that all four patients were able to walk the longest distances while undergoing HBOT, and that they were able to maintain their improvements after the study was over.[40] The authors recommend that HBOT be used until the patient's performance in hyperbaric oxygen does not differ significantly from performance in normal-pressure oxygen or plain air.

When used as an adjunct to surgery, HBOT should be used in ninety-minute sessions at between 2.0 and 2.4 atmospheres absolute. Sessions should be administered twice a day until the patient improves. This may require up to thirty or forty treatments.

We believe that the use of HBOT as an adjunct to various types of surgery is a topic that deserves further research. It is important to note, however, that in cases of sudden and total blockage of a blood vessel, there will not be enough time for HBOT to help new capillaries grow. In such a situation, urgent surgery is often needed, and HBOT should be administered after surgery.

It should also be noted that the patient plays a vital role in PVD treatment. If the patient is a smoker, he or she *must* stop smoking. Any prescribed exercise program should be followed. Risk factors for atherosclerosis must be controlled, which may require weight loss and the taking of prescription medicines, such as those used to reduce high blood pressure. For diabetics, control of the diabetes and proper foot care are both very important. Socks and shoes should not be too tight. The feet should be carefully washed and dried every day, and the skin should be kept soft and dry. Toenails should be properly clipped. Professional treatment is recommended for corns and calluses.

PVD can make life uncomfortable for the patient by producing leg cramps, sores, and cold digits. But more than that, it can be a sign of life-threatening illness. Thus, HBOT can not only make patients with PVD more comfortable, it can possibly help to prolong their lives. In the next chapter, we will look at how HBOT can be used to help prolong the lives of AIDS patients.

CHAPTER 12

Using HBOT
to Treat AIDS

*In Baltimore, 48-year-old Roger J., a steward, is a patient with
AIDS. He has Kaposi's sarcoma, a viral infection that causes purplish skin lesions. Forty lesions cover his face, arms, and legs.
HBOT therapy is started immediately while Roger waits for drug-
treatment approval from his insurance company. For one month,
he receives three one-hour treatments a week. Of the forty lesions,
thirty-four disappear without the drug treatment, which consists
of alpha-interferon injections. HBOT continues after drug treatment begins. All the lesions disappear after three months of
HBOT and alpha-interferon, and the patient gains ten needed
pounds. Roger, who has worn a beard to cover the lesions on his
face, is able to shave. He can go back to work.*

HIV/AIDS is the latest of the world's plagues. About
30 million people worldwide have been infected
with HIV, and about 750,000 million people are living with HIV/AIDS in North America. Millions have died.
Scientists continue to gain a better understanding of HIV
and how it affects the human body. This has led to improvements in treatment. HBOT now plays an important
role in the management of AIDS.

In this chapter, we will first study what HIV/AIDS is,
as well as what complications it can cause. We will then
discuss how HBOT can be used in AIDS treatment. (See

Appendix A for information on contacting hyperbaric oxygen facilities.)

HIV/AIDS AND RELATED COMPLICATIONS

The human immunodeficiency virus (HIV) is passed through sexual contact with an infected person or through contact with infected bodily fluids. It can infect persons of both sexes, including children born to HIV-infected mothers.

HIV causes damage to the immune system and the cardiovascular system. It produces symptoms such as swollen, painful, and tender lymph nodes; a general feeling of malaise; and disabling fatigue. However, HIV may remain in the body for years without causing any symptoms at all.

The rate of progression from the initial HIV infection to fully developed acquired immune deficiency syndrome (AIDS) depends upon the individual; it can take from eighteen months to more than ten years. Women tend to develop AIDS more quickly than men. A patient has AIDS when the level of T-cells, a type of immune-system cell, drops to less than 200 in every milliliter of blood.

Many of the infections associated with HIV result from infections associated with other viruses and bacteria. These infections are called *opportunistic* because, in general, they only affect people with damaged immune systems. There are at least twenty-five opportunistic infections, three of which are:

- Kaposi's sarcoma, a viral infection that may also involve the lymph nodes and other organs

- *Pneumocystis carinii* pneumonia (PCP), a form of pneumonia that generally affects both lungs

- *Mycobacterium avium* complex (MAC), a bacterial infection that causes fever, diarrhea, and abdominal pain; in patients with AIDS, it generally affects organs throughout the body

HIV and its *cofactors* (the viruses that often accompany HIV) also impair the cells that line the blood vessels. This damage can result in blockages of both small and large vessels. These obstructions, in turn, can reduce the flow of blood to the limbs, brain, and heart. Indeed, transient ischemic attacks (TIAs), strokes, and heart attacks are common among patients with AIDS. (A TIA is a short-term stroke; see Chapter 2 for more information.) Daily TIAs increase as the disease progresses, resulting in mental impairment, loss of muscle control, decreased memory, and reduced independence.

HIV/AIDS AND HBOT

Health care practitioners have found HBOT to be useful as part of an overall HIV/AIDS treatment program. HBOT can force oxygen into all of the body's fluids, bypassing the red blood cells, which are the body's regular oxygen carriers. Thus, when blood-vessel complications produce hypoxia, or oxygen starvation in the tissues, HBOT can overcome the hypoxia. HBOT helps reduce the severity of, and secondary complications arising from, opportunistic infections.

The blood-vessel blockages produced by herpes and other viruses have been relieved by HBOT for decades.[1] As we've seen in Chapters 2 and 11, HBOT can aid people with strokes, TIAs, and peripheral vascular disease. So it is not surprising that HBOT can benefit patients with AIDS who experience these problems. HBOT is the recommended therapy for stroke and for peripheral vascular insufficiency, regardless of the underlying disease.

HBOT has improved the lives of many patients with AIDS-related circulation problems. For example, a 29-year-old man had AIDS, but had no HIV/AIDS symptoms and no history of high blood pressure. He suffered a sudden cerebral hemorrhage secondary to an HIV infection of the brain. The cerebral attack left him with left-sided paralysis, and an inability to walk without a walker. The patient started receiving HBOT on a daily basis, for one hour at 2.0 atmospheres absolute (see "The Language of HBOT and of Research" on page 7). He also received physical therapy on an outpatient basis. After two weeks, the patient walked with a cane, again able to use his left leg. He regained his appetite, was relieved of debilitating fatigue, and gained ten pounds. After one month, the patient could lift his left arm, and slowly open and close his left hand. Ongoing HBOT with adjunctive physical therapy enabled the man to resume independent activities with increased mobility.

Kaposi's sarcoma has been linked to one of the many human herpes viruses by Patrick Moore and Yuan Chang.[2] It is an opportunistic viral infection that attacks the blood vessels and causes purplish lesions both externally and internally. It is usually treated with chemotherapy and, often, radiation. HBOT is recommended as an adjunct treatment to reduce the side effects of these therapies in the management of certain cancers.[3] And, as Michelle Reillo has documented in *AIDS Under Pressure* (Hogrefe & Huber, 1997), HBOT is extremely beneficial in the treatment of Kaposi's sarcoma in patients with HIV/AIDS.[4] We saw, in the case study that began this chapter, how HBOT has been used successfully with alpha-interferon injections.

Pneumocystis carinii pneumonia (PCP) kills 60 percent of people with HIV/AIDS despite preventative drug treatment with Bactrim, Dapsone, or aerosol-form pentamidine. HBOT, given three times per week, is an excellent adjunct to preventative drug therapy. Michelle Reillo has found that patients with AIDS who regularly use preventative HBOT and drug therapy develop PCP less often.[5] Additionally, HBOT is recommended in the treatment of acute PCP, along with aggressive chemotherapy.

In one case, a 44-year-old man had acute PCP in both lungs. The patient had lost twenty pounds, was dehydrated and feverish, and was breathing with difficulty. He had been receiving oral Bactrim as a preventative measure. For one hour each day, he received two weeks of HBOT at 2.5 atmospheres absolute, along with intravenous Bactrim. Within five days, his shortness of breath and fevers had gone away. A chest-x-ray revealed complete resolution of the PCP, which had been graded as moderate, within two weeks. The patient also regained ten pounds.

Mycobacterium avium complex (MAC) is an opportunistic infection that can cause organ failure. MAC frequently occurs even in patients who are receiving preventative drug treatment with zithromax, clarithromycin, or rifampin. HBOT, well-documented as an effective adjunctive therapy in tuberculosis caused by *Mycobacterium*, is also effective when used along with drugs in the treatment of MAC. These drugs include the oral therapies ethambutol, zithromax, and ciprofloxin, either alone or when combined with experimental intravenous therapies such as liposomal gentamicin and liposomal amikacin. This has been documented by Michelle Reillo.[6]

In one case, a 39-year-old man had a MAC infection that affected his entire body. The patient had lost thirty pounds, displayed neurologic impairment, had difficulty walking, and had nightly fevers of 101°F. He was taking the standard oral medications, but his weight loss continued. The patient was started on HBOT at 2.5 atmospheres absolute every day for one month, and then three times per week ongoing. After two weeks, his fever and muscle wasting dissipated, and the patient began to eat prepared foods and drink Advera, a liquid supplement. Within one month, the patient gained twenty pounds of healthy weight, and showed improvements in thinking and walking. After two months of treatment, improvement was noted in his mood, motor coordination, and metabolism, and the drug regimen was reduced. Over a two-month period of time, the patient gained twenty-five pounds and showed enough neurologic improvement to operate a computer, which allowed him to resume his work. He continued drug treatment and HBOT.

The dose of HBOT used in the treatment of HIV/AIDS varies from person to person, depending on what specific condition is being treated, how severe the condition is, and what other therapies are being used.

HBOT, when administered as an ongoing treatment, prolongs the quantity and quality of life of people with AIDS, alleviating the blood-vessel problems directly associated with HIV and herpes infections. And, in acute AIDS-related illnesses, HBOT enhances the effectiveness of drug therapies, reduces adverse medication side effects, and shortens the length of life-threatening infections. In the next section, we will look at why HBOT is not employed as often as it can be, and at how it may be used in the future.

Conclusion

After reading this book, you perhaps have decided that HBOT will be able to help you or a loved one overcome a physical problem, such as a stroke, for which your current treatment program is no longer adequate. You may then learn how few hyperbaric chambers there are in the country. You might even call your doctor and find that he or she is unaware of the benefits provided by HBOT.

You could then ask, "If HBOT can be used in so many ways, why haven't I heard of it before? And, more importantly, why hasn't my doctor heard of it?"

There are a number of reasons why this is so, but they fall into three main categories. First, doctors do not know about HBOT because they do not learn about it in medical school. Therefore, they do not prescribe HBOT, which leads to a shortage of hyperbaric chambers. Second, the costs involved in installing and running a chamber can be quite high, although more reasonably priced chambers and simpler installations are becoming available. Third, there is a need for further research in this area.

LACK OF KNOWLEDGE, LACK OF AVAILABILITY

Although modern hyperbaric medicine didn't really develop beyond its underwater beginnings until the 1960s, there is already a massive volume of scientific data on the subject. However, by medical standards, the field is still young. That means there are a lot of doctors who are simply not familiar with HBOT. These doctors are not likely to prescribe a treatment with which they are not familiar.

A good analogy for the way some doctors have responded to HBOT is the way they responded to ulcer research. For years, it was believed that people who developed stomach ulcers were tense, nervous people whose stomachs produced too much acid. Therefore, ulcers were treated with a bland diet and strong antacids. This treatment was not only inappropriate, but caused multiple side effects, including an increased risk of the patient suffering a heart attack. It was then discovered that a bacterial infection was the cause of many ulcers, an infection that could be countered with antibiotics. Yet some doctors continued to prescribe the old treatment regimen. Why? Either they didn't know about the latest in ulcer research—it is not always easy for a busy doctor to keep up with the flood of papers produced each year—or they did not feel that enough research had been done to justify the change in treatment.

American doctors do accept HBOT as a preferred treatment for several conditions. These conditions include poorly healing wounds, chronic bone infections, carbon monoxide poisoning, and air emboli, or air bubbles in the bloodstream (see Chapter 1). Hyperbaric doctors, though, believe that HBOT can be used for many other conditions, including coma resulting from head injuries or near-drowning, bruising of the spinal cord, stroke, and multiple sclerosis. (For a complete list of these conditions, see Appendix B.) It is these additional applications that have yet to be accepted by the medical establishment and the insurance companies.

The situation in the United States stands in marked contrast to the situation in many other countries, where HBOT is used for a much wider range of conditions. In Chapter 4, we saw how multiple sclerosis patients in Great Britain have banded together to create their own network of hyperbaric chambers (see page 50). Centers in China treat more than 90,000 patients each year for a multitude of medical conditions.

Not surprisingly, countries around the world have many more hyperbaric chambers than the United States. There are about 3,000 chambers in Russia, and even more in the other countries that were part of the old Soviet Union. Unfortunately, there are less than 400 chambers in the United States, and they are used to treat only about 100,000 patients a year.

One reason American doctors do not prescribe HBOT as often as their colleagues in other countries is that hyperbaric medicine is not a fully established subject in American medical schools. Hyperbaric chambers are available in fewer than twenty medical schools in the United States. More foreign medical schools have hyperbaric chambers, so these schools are more likely to make hyperbaric medicine part of the curriculum.

Once doctors are out of school, they depend on medical journals and on promotional material from the pharmaceutical industry to keep up with the latest research. But HBOT is not a drug that manufacturers can patent and sell. Therefore, it does not attract the money needed for slick, full-color brochures, or for advertisements in both clinical journals and popular magazines. Doctors, like everyone else, respond to advertising. This means that the only way a doctor can learn about HBOT is by taking the time to research the topic in medical libraries (a task that has become easier since the development of the Internet).

It is important to keep in mind that most hyperbaric doctors are not primary care doctors, and that HBOT is usually not the primary therapy assigned. Hyperbaric doctors are specialists, and thus generally obtain their patients by referral. These referrals mostly come from primary care doctors and from other specialists, such as neurologists. The hyperbaric doctor then consults with the referring doctor and recommends a specific HBOT dosage for that patient. As hyperbaric medicine expands, the hyperbaric doctor will frequently become the primary doctor, provided that the condition under consideration falls into one of the categories for which HBOT is a recognized treatment.

It is also important to remember that doctors who specialize in hyperbaric medicine are practicing in an underutilized field. Thus, there are not as many hyperbaric doctors as there are doctors in other specialized fields, such as orthopedics and internal medicine. In fact, there are fewer than 300 hyperbaric doctors and other personnel in the United States. Therefore, a hyperbaric doctor might not be readily available in any given locality, especially in emergencies.

Indeed, it is in an emergency that the lack of hyperbaric chambers, and of the doctors and other personnel who work with them, presents the biggest problem. For example, there are about 1.5 million heart attack victims each year in the United States. Many of them could be helped by the timely use of HBOT and TPA, a clot-dissolving medicine. With less than 400 hyperbaric oxygen chambers in the country, the chances of a heart attack victim being brought to a hospital with a chamber are not good. And even if the hospital has a chamber, the doctor may not recommend HBOT.

The lack of hyperbaric chambers also affects people with head injuries. Each year, more than 150,000 Americans sustain severe head injuries. A study conducted by the Brain Trauma Foundation, a private organization that finances research on head injuries, showed that many of these people do not receive proper treatment.[1] The foundation learned that most of these patients were improperly monitored, and in some cases, they were treated with ineffective and possibly dangerous methods (see Chapter 3). HBOT is not routinely used, even though we have seen that hyperbaric oxygen can be of enormous benefit for head-injury patients in both the short term and the long term. The absence of HBOT is especially troublesome because the medical care that brain-injured patients receive in the first week after the injury can make the difference between life and death, or between a dependent life and an independent life.

COST OF CHAMBERS VERSUS
COST OF TREATMENT

Cost is part of the reason hyperbaric chambers are not standard equipment at hospitals and medical centers. Monoplace chambers range in price from $80,000 to $150,000. Multiplace chambers vary in cost according to size. A four-person multiplace chamber may be purchased for about $250,000, including the compressor and all other necessary equipment, while costs for larger chambers may run into millions of dollars.

Hyperbaric chambers also require trained operating personnel, especially the larger multiplace chambers. Also, use of the larger chambers requires adherence to the strict requirements of the U.S. Occupational Safety and Health Administration (OSHA). These requirements help safeguard both operators and patients, but do add to a chamber's operating costs.

Cost by itself, however, need not be a deterrent to the wide use of any piece of equipment. For example, magnetic resonance imaging (MRI) scanners are also expensive. They cost between $750,000 and $1.7 million a unit (installed), depending on the type of unit purchased. And a million-dollar unit costs about $1.3 million to operate each year. Despite the cost, MRI is used constantly because it has proven to be a valuable diagnostic tool. Thus, a number of hospitals and freestanding clinics have invested in MRI scanners, as these organizations know that their expenses will be more than offset by their income.

One reason cost has not been a deterrent to the availability of MRI technology is that third-party payers, such as insurance companies, will pay for it. They pay because they see MRI as being useful in a large number of situations. Quite differently, there is limited third-party reimbursement for HBOT because third-party payers have not recognized that HBOT is very cost effective, especially when provided in an outpatient facility rather than a hospital. Third-party payers will pay for HBOT in little more than a dozen situations. If hyperbaric chambers are accepted as wholeheartedly as MRI scanners have been, there will be more third-party reimbursement for HBOT. At that point, hyperbaric chambers will be seen as a reasonable investment, and therefore will be more readily available. We believe this scenario might come about if the managed-care industry takes a close look at HBOT.

MRI scanners and hyperbaric chambers have something else in common. It is more expensive to undergo an MRI scan than it is to have an x-ray taken. However, the MRI can give the doctor a much more detailed look at what is happening within the patient without the need for exploratory surgery. In most cases, the extra information, gained at relatively little risk to the patient, is well worth the extra cost.

In a similar fashion, HBOT can be more expensive on a per-usage basis than other treatments, such as drugs. However, HBOT's cost is outweighed by its benefits:

- *HBOT is noninvasive.* It does not involve entering the patient's body. This is important because patients who receive HBOT are generally undergoing other, more invasive procedures, such as surgery.

- *HBOT is safe.* Unlike many other treatments, HBOT has few side effects, and almost none of any lasting nature (see Chapter 1).

- *HBOT works well with other treatments.* As we've seen in previous chapters, HBOT can be used to make various other forms of treatment more effective. Its lack of side effects means that a doctor doesn't have to worry about what complications may arise as a result of HBOT and another treatment being used together.

In the long run, HBOT may even be cheaper than other

forms of treatment. With a few exceptions, patients receive HBOT for a fixed number of sessions, and the treatment tends to be definitive—either it helps the patient or it doesn't. Now, a patient may take a certain drug for a very long period of time, perhaps for a lifetime. At some point, the cost of medication may well exceed the cost of HBOT. That is especially true if the medication used does not overcome the condition being treated, but only keeps it in check—which means a maintenance level of healing, not a definitive cure. In addition, the patient may develop a tolerance for a particular drug, in which case larger and larger dosages are required to elicit a response.

HBOT can also be cheaper in the long run because it can speed up the healing process. For example, the normal expenditure involved in the effort to heal a fracture nonunion (see Chapter 8) without the use of HBOT can be in excess of $250,000. With HBOT, it can cost less than $25,000. HBOT could also be used to accelerate wound healing. Such usage could, in a well-selected majority of cases, shorten the recovery time by 20 to 40 percent. The equipment needed to accomplish this would cost less than $200 million, whereas the money saved in the use of hospital beds alone could exceed $10 billion a year.

FUTURE STUDIES WITH HBOT

There are about 20,000 papers on the use of HBOT from researchers around the world, and the list keeps growing. Ongoing research occurs in every field of medicine, and hyperbaric medicine is no exception.

Not all these studies have shown positive results. For example, we mentioned a study in Chapter 3 in which dogs with brain damage resulting from cardiac arrest were not helped by one session of HBOT.[2] This result is not at all surprising. No one, including these authors, would expect one session to overcome any condition. In some studies involving human patients, HBOT did not bring about the desired results. This is also not surprising. As we hope we've made clear, HBOT is not a magical cure-all. HBOT is a very useful treatment, but like all treatments, it has its limits. The patient's age and overall physical condition, along with the severity of his or her disease or injury, must be taken into account. Not every patient will have a positive response.

It must be said that, in many cases of HBOT failure, HBOT was the treatment of last resort. All other possible treatments had been tried before HBOT, and all had failed. Unfortunately, hyperbaric medicine's critics will often point at these failures and say, "We knew it wouldn't work." It is important for both doctors and patients to understand that, as with all treatments, HBOT is more effective when used in a timely manner.

You should keep something in mind when you read about medical studies. In the medical research of any field, it is important that a proper *protocol* be followed. A protocol is a plan of treatment that researchers follow when they conduct a study. For a study on HBOT, a protocol would specify, among other things, the pressure to be used, the amount of time for each session, and the total number of sessions. When following up on original research, scientists must adhere to the protocol used in the original study. In the case of HBOT, this has not always been the case. It appears that self-defeating protocols—protocols that are inappropriate for the condition being treated—have been used to ensure negative results by those who oppose the use of HBOT.

Good protocols are important, because doctors still want to explore a number of issues in hyperbaric medicine. We believe that the greatest potential benefit of HBOT lies in the fields of cardiology and neurology. There is strong evidence that HBOT can help save heart-attack victims. Studies are needed to ascertain HBOT's role in cardiology as a whole.

Studies are now being designed to evaluate HBOT in cases of acute stroke. It has been suggested that ambulances in the United States, like those in Japan, be equipped with portable hyperbaric bags. Such bags would allow patients suffering from strokes, heart attacks, near-drownings, and other emergency conditions to receive pressurized oxygen on the way to the hospital. Also, many hospitals are now getting together to use a specific HBOT protocol for acute stroke within the first three hours, both with and without TPA.

Studies are also continuing involving the SPECT imaging system (see Chapter 2), together with HBOT, to predict how much brain function can be recovered after a stroke or other types of brain injury. As these studies continue to show positive results, it may be possible to send some stroke patients home from the hospital and avoid nursing-home care. Treating them as outpatients with HBOT and physical therapy could produce savings that would be in the billions of dollars.

Public education on HBOT and stroke needs to be improved. Many strokes occur at night. Unfortunately, many patients do not want to bother their doctors in the middle of the night, or will call and be referred to an MRI center and a neurologist. Under these circumstances, up to twenty-four hours may elapse before the patient actually receives treatment. As we saw in Chapter 2, HBOT is most effective when used as soon after the stroke occurs as possible. That's why doctors have started calling strokes "brain attacks," similar to heart attacks, to draw the public's attention to the need for immediate treatment. Research and education must go hand in hand.

We believe that, as more doctors learn about the benefits of HBOT, more of them will make use of this highly effective treatment method. HBOT will then assume a larger role in the practice of medicine. We hope this book will stimulate readers to discuss hyperbaric medicine with their friends, doctors, and local hospitals, so that many more HBOT centers will become available. Medical science stands on the brink of seeing a twentieth-century treatment become a twenty-first-century boon to healing. HBOT has that kind of potential. What is needed to make this happen? More research but, more than that, an educated public that demands access to this safe, noninvasive therapy. We hope this book is a step in the right direction.

APPENDIX A

Contacting Hyperbaric Oxygen Facilities

Some hyperbaric medicine organizations and facilities are listed below. For information on a chamber in your area, contact either the American College of Hyperbaric Medicine (via the Ocean Hyperbaric Center) or the Undersea Hyperbaric Medical Society.

**American College of
  Hyperbaric Medicine**
See Ocean Hyperbaric Center

Baptist Medical Center
800 Prudential Drive
Jacksonville FL 32207
904-202-1151

Lifeforce
1006 Morton Street, Suite 100
Baltimore MD 21201
410-528-0150

Ocean Hyperbaric Center
4001 Ocean Drive
Lauderdale-by-the-Sea FL 33308
954-771-4000
Fax: 954-776-0670

E-mail: taamb@aol.com
Website: http://www.Hyper-baric-oxygen.com

**Texas A&M University
  Hyperbaric Laboratory**
A.P. Beutel Health Center
College Station TX 77843-1264
409-845-5031

**Undersea Hyperbaric Medical
  Society Inc.**
10531 Metropolitan Avenue
Kensington MD 20895-2627
301-942-2980
Fax: 301-942-7804
E-mail: uhms@radix.net
Website: http://www.umhs.org

For further study, you may want to consult the following books:

AIDS Under Pressure by Michelle Reillo (Kirkland WA: Hogrefe & Huber, 1997, 206-820-1500/800-228-3749).

Hyperbaric Medicine Procedures by E.P. Kindwall and R.W. Goldman (Milwaukee WI: St. Luke's Hospital, 1988).
Textbook of Hyperbaric Medicine by K.K. Jain, M.D. (Toronto: Hogrefe & Huber, 1996).

List of Conditions That Have Been Treated With HBOT

This is a list of conditions that have been treated with HBOT. In many instances, further longitudinal double-blind controlled studies are indicated. It is from a clinical stand-point that the following conditions may well benefit from hyperbaric oxygen, especially when other measures have failed.

Emergency Indications

Air embolism

Decompression sickness

Burns

Carbon monoxide poisoning

Cerebral edema

Closed head injuries

Crisis of sickle cell anemia

Blast injury

Gas gangrene

Hydrogen sulfide poisoning

Near-drowning

Near-electrocution

Near-hanging

Peyote poisoning

Severed limbs

Smoke inhalation

Ileus

Specific Neurologic Indications

Air embolism
   a. Decompression induced
   b. Iatrogenic

Cerebral edema
   a. Toxic encephalopathy
   b. Vasogenic
   c. Traumatic

Spinal cord contusion
   a. Physiological transection
   b. Partial motor or sensory loss

Early organic brain syndrome
a. Small vessel disease

Stroke
a. Acute
b. Chronic

Vegetative coma
a. Closed head injury
b. Hypoxic encephalopathy

Multiple sclerosis
a. Acute
b. Relapsing/remitting
c. Chronic progressive

Cranial nerve syndromes
a. Trigeminal neuralgia
b. Optic neuritis
c. Vestibular disorders
d. Sudden deafness
e. Brain stem syndromes
f. Retinal artery occlusion

Peripheral neuropathy
a. Charcot Marie's tooth disease
b. Radiation myelitis

Orthopedic Indications

Crush injuries

Soft tissue swelling
a. Traumatic
b. Cellulitis (infection/mixed flora)

Compartment syndrome

Acute necrotizing fasciitis

Clostridial myonecrosis

Severed limbs and digits

Acute and chronic osteomyelitis

Bone grafting

Fracture nonunion

Aseptic necrosis

Tendon and ligament injuries, post-surgical repair

Delayed wound healing

Stump infections

Edema under cast

Miscellaneous Indications

Peripheral vascular ulcer
a. Arterial
b. Decubitus
c. Neuropathy related
d. Venous

Gangrene (wet and dry)

Buerger's disease

Frostbite

Diabetic retinopathy

Retinal artery occlusion

Retinal vein thrombosis

Lepromatous leprosy

Migraine

Pneumatosis cystoides intestinalis

Pseudomembranous colitis

Rheumatoid arthritis (acute), scleroderma

Sickle cell crisis and hematuria

Peptic ulcer

Myocardial infarction

Post-cardiotomy low output failure

Radiation cystitis and enteritis

Refractory mycoses

Chronic fatigue

Cerebral palsy

Post-polio syndrome

Cirrhosis

Crohn's disease

Notes

Guide to Abbreviations

Acta Chirurg Scand   Acta Chirurgica Scandinavia
Acta Neurochir   Acta Neurochirgica
Acta Physiol Scand   Acta Physiologica Scandinavica
Adv Exp Med Biol   Advances in Experimental Medicine
and Biology
Aerosp Med   Aerospace Medicine
Am J Dis Child   American Journal of the Disabled Child
Am J Emer Med   American Journal of Emergency
Medicine
Am J Surg   American Journal of Surgery
Am Surgeon   American Surgeon
Ann Emer Med   Annals of Emergency Medicine
Ann Intern Med   Annals of Internal Medicine
Ann Neurol   Annals of Neurology
Ann NY Acad Sci   Annals of the New York Academy of
Sciences
Ann Otol Rhinol Laryngol   Annals of Otology, Rhinology,
and Laryngology
Ann Plast Surg   Annals of Plastic Surgery
Ann R Coll Surg Engl   Annals of the Royal College of
Surgeons of England

Ann Rev Microbiol   Annual Review of Microbiology
Antonie Leeuwenhoek Microbiol   Antonie van Leeuwenhoek
   Microbiologie
Arch Chirurg Neederlandic   Archiva Chirurgica
   Neederlandic
Arch Chirurg Scand   Archiva Chirurgica Scandinavica
Arch Neurol   Archives of Neurology
Arch Otorhinolaryngol   Archives of Otorhinolaryngology
Aust NZ J Med   Australian and New Zealand Journal of
   Medicine
Aviat Space Environ Med   Aviation, Space, and
   Environmental Medicine

BMJ   British Medical Journal
Br J Med   British Journal of Medicine
Br J Radiol   British Journal of Radiology
Br J Surg   British Journal of Surgery

Cardio J of Microbiol   Cardiology Journal of Microbiology
Cardiovasc Clin   Cardiovascular Clinics
Clin Orthop   Clinical Orthopedics
Clin Ped   Clinical Pediatrics
Clin Toxicol   Clinical Toxicology
Contemp Ortho   Contemporary Orthopedics
Curr Con Wound Care   Current Concepts in Wound Care

Dan Med Bull   Danish Medical Bulletin

Emer Clin North Am   Emergency Medicine Clinics of
   North America
Emer Med   Emergency Medicine
Eur Neurol   European Neurology

Handchir Mikrochir Plast Chir   Handchirugie,
   Mikrochirugie, Plastiche Chirugie

Igaku Jpn   Igaku Japan
Int Angiol   International Angiology

Int J Radiat Oncol Bio Phys   International Journal of
  Radiation Oncology, Biology, and Physics
Int Med   Internal Medicine

J Am Dent Assoc   Journal of the American Dental
  Association
J Bacteriol   Journal of Bacteriology
J Bone Joint Surg   Journal of Bone and Joint Surgery
J Clin Path   Journal of Clinical Pathology
J Emer Med   Journal of Emergency Medicine
J Hyper Med   Journal of Hyperbaric Medicine
J Ind Hyg Toxicol   Journal of Industrial Hygiene and
  Toxicology
J Infect Dis   Journal of Infectious Diseases
J Mal Vasc   Journal des Maladies Vasulares
J Mt Sinai Hosp   Journal of Mount Sinai Hospital
J Neurol   Journal of Neurology
J Neurol Neurosug Psychiatry   Journal of Neurology,
  Neurosurgery, and Psychiatry
J Neurosurg   Journal of Neurosurgery
J Nucl Med   Journal of Nuclear Medicine
J Ortho Res   Journal of Orthopaedic Research
J Pharmacol Exp Ther   Journal of Pharmacology and
  Experimental Therapy
J Physiol   Journal of Physiology
J Roy Soc Med   Journal of the Royal Society of Medicine
J Surg Res   Journal of Surgical Research
J Thorac Cardiovasc Surg   Journal of Thoratic and
  Cardiovascular Surgery
J Trauma   Journal of Trauma
J Urol   Journal of Urology
JAMA   Journal of the American Medical Association
Jpn J Hyperbaric Med   Japanese Journal of Hyperbaric
  Medicine

Med Hypotheses   Medical Hypotheses
Med Subacquea ed Iperbarica Minerva Med   Medica
  Subacquea ed Iperbarica Minerva Medica

Mich Med   Michigan Medicine
Mil Med   Military Medicine
Minn Med   Minnesota Medicine

N Eng J Med   New England Journal of Medicine
Neurochem Res   Neurochemical Research
NY State J Med   New York State Journal of Medicine

Plast Reconstr Surg   Plastic and Reconstructive Surgery
Postgrad Med J   Postgraduate Medical Journal
Pre Med   Preventative Medicine
Psych Neurol Scand   Psychologie et Neurologie
   Scandinavica

Revist de Leprologica   Revista Brasieira de Leprologica
Roche Med Image Commentary   Roche Medical Image and
   Commentary

Semin Hematol   Seminars in Hematology
Soviet Med   Soviet Medicine
Surg Forum   Surgical Forum
Surg Gynecol Obstet   Surgery, Gynecology, and Obstetrics
Surg Neurol   Surgical Neurology
Surg Rounds   Surgical Rounds

Trans Royal Soc Edinb   Transactions of the Royal Society
   of Edinborogh
Traumas Arch Otorhinolaryngol   Trauma Archiva
   Otorhinolaryngolie
Top Emer Med   Topics in Emergency Medicine
Toxicol Appl Pharmacol   Toxicology and Applied
   Pharmacology

Undersea Biomed Res   Undersea Biomedical Research

Zh Neuropatol Psikhiatr   Zhurnal Neuropatologgi i
   Psikhiatrii

Chapter 1
Oxygen Under Pressure:
Hyperbaric Oxygen Therapy
1. Sukoff M.H. and Gottlieb S.F. Hyperbaric oxygen therapy. In Nussbaum E. (ed): *Pediatric Intensive Care*. 2nd ed. Mount Kisco, New York: Futura Publishing Inc., 1989, pp. 483–507.
2. Neubauer R.A., Kagan R.L., and Gottlieb S.F. Use of hyperbaric oxygen for the treatment of aseptic bone necrosis. *J Hyper Med* 4:69–76, 1989.
3. Gottlieb S.F. Proposed criteria for evaluating disease entities for inclusion in accepted indications category for hyperbaric oxygen treatment. *J Hyper Med* 4:33–37, 1989.
4. Gottlieb S.F. and Neubauer R.A. Multiple sclerosis: its etiology, pathogenesis, and therapeutics with emphasis on the controversial use of HBO. *J Hyper Med* 5:143–164, 1988.
5. Gilbert D.L. Perspective on the history of oxygen and life. In Gilbert D.L. (ed): *Oxygen and Living Processes: An Interdisciplinary Approach*. New York: Springer-Verlag, 1981, pp. 1–43.
6. Gilbert D.L. Significance of oxygen on earth. In Gilbert D.L. (ed): *Oxygen and Living Processes: An Interdisciplinary Approach*. New York: Springer-Verlag, 1981, pp. 73–101.
7. Davis J.C. and Hunt T.K. (eds). *Hyperbaric Oxygen Therapy*. Bethesda, Maryland: Undersea Medical Society, 1977, pp. xi–xii.
8. Sukoff M.H. and Gottlieb S.F. Hyperbaric oxygen therapy. In Nussbaum E. (ed): *Pediatric Intensive Care*. 2nd ed. Mount Kisco, New York: Futura Publishing Inc., 1989, pp. 483–507.
9. Jacobson J.H. II, Morsch J.H.C., and Rendell-Baker L. The historical perspective of hyperbaric therapy. *Ann NY Acad Sci* 117:651–670, 1965.
10. Armstrong D. The Trulocks: a story of love, frustration and perseverance . . .. *The Dixon Telegraph*, 10/15/91, p. 1.

Chapter 2
Using HBOT to Treat Stroke
1. Jain K.K. *Cerebral Insufficiency*. Chicago: Year Book Medical Publishers, 1990.
2. Astrup J., Siesjo B.K., and Symon L. Thresholds in cerebral ischemia, the ischemic penumbra. *Stroke* 12:723, 1981.
3. Simon L. The concept of threshold of ischemia in relation to brain structure and function. *J Clin Path* 11(suppl): 149–154, 1976.
4. Astrup J., Siesjo B.K., and Symon L. The state of penumbra in the ischemic brain: viable and lethal threshold in cerebral ischemia. *Stroke* 12:723–725, 1981.
5. Neubauer R.A., Kagan R.L., Gottlieb S.F., and James P.B. Letter. *Lancet*, 3 March 1990.
6. Neubauer R.A., Gottlieb S.F., and Kagan R.L. Enhancing "idling" neurons. *Lancet* 335:542, 1990.
7. Neubauer R.A. The effect of hyperbaric oxygen in prolonged coma. Possible identification of marginal functioning brain zones. *Med Subacquea ed Iperbarica Minerva Med* 5(3):75–79, 1985.
8. Boerema I., Meyne N.G., Brummelkamp W.H., and others. Life without blood. *Arch Chirurg Nee-*

derlandic 11:70–83, 1959.

9. Neubauer R.A. and Gottlieb S.F. Stroke treatment. *Lancet* 337:1601, 1991.

10. Kaasik A.E., Dimitriev K.K., and Tomberg T.A. Hyperbaric oxygenation in the treatment of patients with ischemic stroke. *Zh Nevropatol Psikhiatr* 88:38–43, 1988.

11. Smith G., Lawson D.D., Renfrew S., and others. Preservation of cerebral cortical activity by breathing oxygen at 2 ATA pressure during cerebral ischemia. *Surg Gynecol Obstet* 113: 13, 1961.

12. Whalen R., Heyman A., and Saltzman H. The protective effect of hyperbaric oxygen in cerebral ischemia. *Arch Neurol* 14:15, 1966.

13. Moore G.F., Fuson R.L., Margolis G., and others. An evaluation of the protective effect of hyperbaric oxygenation on the central nervous system during circulatory arrest. *J Thorac Cardiovasc Surg* 52:618, 1966.

14. Corkill G., Dhousen K., Hein H., and others. Videodensimetric estimation of the protective effect of hyperbaric oxygen in the ischemic gerbil brain. *Surg Neurol* 24:406, 1985.

15. Shiokawa D., Fujishima M., Yanai T., and others. Hyperbaric oxygen therapy in experimentally induced acute cerebral ischemia. *Undersea Biomed Res* 13:337, 1986.

16. Burt J.T., Kapp J.P., and Smith R.R. Hyperbaric oxygen and cerebral infarction in the gerbil. *Surg Gynecol* 28:265, 1987.

17. Weinstein P.R., Hameroff S.R., Johnson P., and others. Effect of hyperbaric oxygen therapy or dimethylsulfoxide on cerebral ischemia in unanesthetized gerbils. *Neurosurgery* 18:528, 1986.

18. Reiten J.A., Kien N.D., Thorup S., and others. Hyperbaric oxygen increases survival following carotid ligation in gerbils. *Stroke* 21:119–123, 1990.

19. Jacobson I. and Lawson D.D. The effect of hyperbaric oxygen on experimental cerebral infarction in the dog. *J Neurosurg* 20: 849, 1963.

20. Holbach K.H., Wassmann H., Hoheluchter K.L., and Jain K.K. Differentiation between reversible and irreversible poststroke changes in brain tissue. *Surg Neurol* 7:325, 1977.

21. Neubauer R.A. and End E. Hyperbaric oxygenation as an adjunct therapy in strokes due to thrombosis. *Stroke* 11:297–300, 1980.

22. Jain K.K. Effect of hyperbaric oxygenation on spasticity in stroke patients. *J Hyper Med* 4: 55–61, 1989.

23. Mountz J.M., Modell J.G., Foster N.L., and others. Prognostication of recovery following stroke using the comparison of CT and technetium-99 HMPAO SPECT. *J Nucl Med* 31:6–66, 1990.

24. Neubauer R.A., Kagan R.L., Gottlieb S.F., and James P.B. Letter. *Lancet*, 3 March 1990.

25. Neubauer R.A., Gottlieb S.F., and Kagan R.L. Enhancing "idling" neurons. *Lancet* 335:542, 1990.

Chapter 3
Using HBOT to Treat Central Nervous System and Sensory Problems

1. Jain K.K., ed. *Textbook of Hyperbaric Medicine.* Toronto: Hogrefe & Huber, 1990.
2. Jain K.K. *Oxygen in Physiology and Medicine.* Springfield, Illinois: Charles C. Thomas, 1989.
3. DeVolder A.G., Goffinet A.M., Bol A., and others. Brain glucose metabolism in postanoxic syndrome. *Arch Neurol* 47:197–204, 1990.
4. Kolata G. Flawed treatment of head injuries found. *The New York Times,* 10/16/91, p. C14.
5. Mathieu D., Wattel F., Gosselin B., and others. Hyperbaric oxygen in the treatment of posthanging cerebral anoxia. *J Hyper Med* 2:63–67, 1987.
6. Plum F. and Posner J.B. The diagnosis of stupor and coma. *Edition* 3:338–340, 1981.
7. Coe J.E. and Hayes T.M. Treatment of experimental brain injury by hyperbaric oxygen. Preliminary report. *Am Surgeon* 32: 493, 1966.
8. Fasano V.A., Nunno T., Urciuoli R., and others. First observations on the use of oxygen under high atmospheric pressure for treatment of traumatic coma. In Boerema I., Brummelkamp W.H., and Meijne N.G. (eds): *Clinical Applications of Hyperbaric Oxygen. Proceedings of the First International Congress on Hyperbaric Medicine.* Amsterdam: Elsevier, 1964, pp. 168–173.
9. Neubauer R.A. The effect of hyperbaric oxygen in prolonged coma. Possible identification of marginally functioning brain zones. *Med Subacquea ed Iperbarica Minerva Med* 5(3):75–79, 1985.
10. Neubauer R.A. Hyperbaric oxygen in vegetative coma. In Schutz J. (ed): *Proceedings of the First Swiss Symposium on Hyperbaric Medicine.* Basel, Switzerland: Foundation for Hyperbaric Medicine, 1986, p. 116.
11. BeLokurov M.I., Stephaokov A.A., and Kirsanov B.I. Hyperbaric oxygenation in the combined therapy of comatose states in children. *Pediatrtia* 2: 84–87, 1988.
12. Ruiz E., Brunette D.D., Robinson E.P., and others. Cerebral resuscitation after cardiac arrest using hetasterch hemodilution, hyperbaric oxygenation, and magnesium ion. *Resuscitation* 14:213–223, 1986.
13. Holbach K.H., Wassmann H., and Kolberg T. Verbesserte reversibilatat des traumatischen mittelhirnsyndrome bei anwendung der hyperbaren oxygenierung. [Improved reversal of traumatic-brain syndrome by application of hyperbaric oxygen.] *Acta Neurochir* 30:247–256, 1974.
14. Holbach K.H., Caroli A., and Wassmann H. Cerebral energy metabolism in patients with brain lesions at normo- and hyperbaric oxygen pressure. *J Neurol* 217:17–30, 1977.
15. Jain K.K., ed. *Textbook of Hyperbaric Medicine.* Toronto: Hogrefe & Huber, 1990.
16. Mogami H., Hayakawa T., Kanal N., and others. Clinical application of hyperbaric oxygenation in the treatment of acute cerebral damage. *J Neurosurg* 31:636–643, 1969.

17. Holbach K.H., Wassmann H., and Kolberg T. Verbesserte reversibilatat des traumatischen mittelhirnsyndrome bei anwendung der hyperbaren oxygenierung. [Improved reversal of traumatic-brain syndrome by application of hyperbaric oxygen.] *Acta Neurochir* 30:247–256, 1974.

18. Artu F., Philippon B., Gau F., Berger M., and Deleuze R. Cerebral blood flow, cerebral metabolism and cerebrospinal fluid biochemistry in brain-injured patients after exposure to hyperbaric oxygen. *Eur Neurol* 14:351–364, 1976.

19. Sukoff M.H. and Ragatz R.E. Hyperbaric oxygenation for the treatment of acute cerebral edema. *Neurosurgery* 10:29–38, 1982.

20. Rockswold G.L. and Ford S.E. Preliminary results of a prospective randomized trial for treatment of severely brain-injured patients with hyperbaric oxygen. *Minn Med* 68:533–535, 1985.

21. Gelderd J.B., Welch D.W., Fife W.P., and Bowers D.E. Therapeutic effects of hyperbaric oxygen and dimethyl sulfoxide following spinal cord transections in rats. *Undersea Biomed Res 7* (4):305–320, 1980.

22. Neretin V.I., Kirjakov V.A., Lobov M.A., and Kiselev S.O. Hyperbaric oxygenation in dyscirculatory myelopathies. *Soviet Medicine* 3:42–44, 1985.

23. Kieper N.R. The use of hyperbaric oxygen in the rehabilitation of spinal cord injured patients due to decompression sickness. In Kindwall E.P. (ed): *Proceedings of the Eighth International Congress on Hyperbaric Medicine*. San Pedro, California: Best, 1987.

24. Dalessio D.A. Complexity of headaches. *Emer Med* 4:25–64, 1981.

25. Olsen J., Larsen B., and Lauritzen M. Focal hyperemia followed by spreading oligemia and impaired activation of rCBF in classical migraine. *Ann Neurol* 9:344–352, 1981.

26. Meyer J.S. Regulation of cerebral hemodynamics in health and disease. *Eur Neurol* 22(1):47–60, 1983.

27. Amery W.K. Brain hypoxia: the turning-point in the genesis of the migraine attack? *Cephalalgia* 2:83–109, 1982.

28. Fife W.P. and Fife C.E. Treatment of migraine with hyperbaric oxygen. *J Hyper Med* 4(1):7–15, 1989.

29. Sukoff M.H. and Ragatz R.E. Hyperbaric oxygenation for the treatment of acute cerebral edema. *Neurosurgery* 10:29–38, 1982.

30. Rockswold G.L. and Ford S.E. Preliminary results of a prospective randomized trial for treatment of severely brain-injured patients with hyperbaric oxygen. *Minn Med* 68:533–535, 1985.

31. Sukoff M. Central nervous system: review and update on cerebral edema and spinal cord injuries. *HBO Review* 1:189–195, 1980.

32. Pilgramm M., Lamm H., and Jain K.K. Hyperbaric oxygen therapy in otolaryngology. In Jain K.K. (ed): *Textbook of Hyperbaric Medicine*. Toronto: Hogrefe & Huber, 1996, p. 405.

33. Pilgramm M., Lamm H., and

Jain K.K. Hyperbaric oxygen therapy in otolaryngology. In Jain K.K. (ed): *Textbook of Hyperbaric Medicine.* Toronto: Hogrefe & Huber, 1996, p. 406.

34. Eibach H. and Börger U. Therapeutische Ergebnisse in der Behandlung des akuten akustichen Traumas. [Therapeutic results in the handling of acute acoustic trauma.] *Arch Otorhinolaryngol* 226:177–186, 1980.

35. Beck C. Pathologie der innenohrscghwerhorigkeit. [Pathology of inner ear hearing loss.] *Arch Orh Nas Kehl Heilk* 1(Suppl):1–57, 1984.

36. Lamm C.H., Walliser U., Schumann K., and Lamm K. Sauerstoffpartialdruck Messungen in der Perilymphe der Scala tympani unter normo- und hyperbaren Bedingungen. [Oxygen partial pressure in the perilymph of the scala tympani under normo- and hyperbaric conditions.] *HNO* 36:363–366, 1988.

37. Matthieu D., Coget J., Vinchkier I., and others. Red blood cell deformity and hyperbaric oxygenation. In: *Proceedings of the Eighth International Congress on Hyperbaric Medicine.* Long Beach, California: Long Beach Memorial Hospital, 1984, pp. 27–28.

38. Lamm H. Klinische Ergebnisse nach Behandlung von Innenohrschwerhörigkeiten mit hyperbarem Saurstoff. [Results and conditions of inner-ear hearing loss with hyperbaric oxgyen.] *Diskuss.* Halle/Saale: Beitrag HNO-Jahrekongress der DDR, 1969.

39. Yefuni S.N., Levashova A.S., and Lyskin G.I. Hyperbaric oxygenation in the treatment of the cochleovestibular system. *Soviet Med* 5:45–49, 1980.

40. Lyskin G.I. and Levashova A.S. Hyperbaric oxygenation in the treatment of labyrinthopathies of vascular genesis. In Yefuni S.N. (ed): *Abstracts of the Seventh International Congress of Hyperbaric Medicine.* Moscow: USSR Academy of Sciences, 1981, p. 307.

41. Kosyro V.I. and Matskevich M.V. Clinical aspects of using hyperbaric oxygenation in the treatment of different forms of neurosensory hypoacusis. In Yefuni S.N. (ed): *Abstracts of the Seventh International Congress of Hyperbaric Medicine.* Moscow: USSR Academy of Sciences, 1981, pp. 306–307.

42. Pilgramm M., Lamm H., and Jain K.K. Hyperbaric oxygen therapy in otolaryngology. In Jain K.K. (ed): *Textbook of Hyperbaric Medicine.* Toronto: Hogrefe & Huber, 1996, p. 411.

43. Pilgramm M., Lamm H., and Jain K.K. Hyperbaric oxygen therapy in otolaryngology. In Jain K.K. (ed): *Textbook of Hyperbaric Medicine.* Toronto: Hogrefe & Huber, 1996, p. 407.

44. Bojic L., Gosovic S., Kovacecic H., and Denoble P. *Hyperbaric Oxygenation in the Treatment of Macular Degeneration.* Split, Yugoslavia: Split Naval Medical Institute, pp. 1–4.

Chapter 4
Using HBOT to Treat Multiple Sclerosis

1. Lumsden C.E. The neuropathology of multiple sclero-

sis: multiple sclerosis and other demyelinating diseases. In Vinken P. and Bruyn G.W. (eds): *Handbook of Clinical Neurology.* Vol. 9. Amsterdam: North Holland Publishing, 1970, pp. 217–309.

2. Dawson J.W. The histology of disseminated sclerosis. *Trans Royal Soc Edinb* 1(3):517–540, 1916.

3. Pollock M., Calder C., and Alpress S. Peripheral nerve abnormality in multiple sclerosis. *Ann Neurol* 2:41–48, 1977.

4. Hart M. Periphlebitis retinae in association with multiple sclerosis. *Psych Neurol Scand* 29: 175–189, 1953.

5. Aita J.F., Bennett D.R., Anderson R.E., and Ziter F. Cranial CT appearance of acute multiple sclerosis. *Neurology* 28:251–255, 1928.

6. Swank R.L. Subcutaneous hemorrhages in multiple sclerosis. *Neurology* 8:497–499, 1958.

7. Dow R.S. and Berglund G. Vascular pattern of lesions of multiple sclerosis. *Arch Neurol* 47:1–18, 1942.

8. Brownell B. and Hughes J.T. The distribution of plaques in the cerebrum in multiple sclerosis. *J Neurol Neurosurg Psychiatry* 25:315–320, 1962.

9. Chattaway S.J.S. What's new in the pathogenesis of multiple sclerosis? A review. *J Roy Soc Med* 82:159–162, 1989.

10. Gottlieb S.F. and Neubauer R.A. Multiple sclerosis: its etiology, pathogenesis, and therapeutics with emphasis on the controversial use of HBO. *J Hyper Med* 3:143–164, 1988.

11. McDonald W.I. The mystery of the origin of multiple sclerosis. *J Neurol Neurosurg Psychiatry* 49:113–123, 1986.

12. Weiner H.L. COP 1 therapy for multiple sclerosis. *N Eng J Med* 317:442–444, 1987.

13. Cook S.D. and Dowling P.C. Multiple sclerosis and viruses: an overview. *Neurobiology* 30: 80–91, 1980.

14. Wolfgram F. What if multiple sclerosis isn't an immunological or a viral disease? The case for a circulating toxin. *Neurochem Res* 4:1–4, 1979.

15. James P.B. Evidence for subacute fat embolism as the cause of multiple sclerosis. *Lancet* 1:380–385, 1982.

16. Wolfgram F. What if multiple sclerosis isn't an immunological or a viral disease? The case for a circulating toxin. *Neurochem Res* 4:1–4, 1979.

17. Stein E.C., Schiffer R.B., Jackson W., and Young N. Multiple sclerosis and the work place: report of an industry-based cluster. *Neurology* 37:1672–1677, 1987.

18. Gottlieb S.F. and Neubauer R.A. The etiology of multiple sclerosis: a new and extended vascular-ischemic model. *Med Hypotheses* 33:23–29, 1990.

19. Field E.J. Letter to the editor. *Lancet* 1:1273, 1989.

20. James P.B. Letter to the editor. *Lancet* 1:1273, 1989.

21. Simpson L.O. Letter to the editor. *Lancet* 1:1272–1273, 1989.

22. Gottlieb S.F. and Neubauer R.A. Multiple sclerosis: its etiology, pathogenesis, and therapeutics with emphasis on the controversial use of HBO. *J Hyper Med* 3:143–164, 1988.

23. Poulton G.A. Controversial MS treatment provides degree

of help and hope for victims. *Fort Lauderdale News* 8/9/82, p 2B.

24. Haney D.Q. MS victims find hope in treatment. *The Philadelphia Inquirer* 9/25/83, pp. 1-C, 8-C.

25. Fischer B.H., Marks M., and Reich T. Hyperbaric-oxygen treatment of multiple sclerosis. *N Engl J Med* 308 (4):181–186, 1983.

26. Yamada T., Hirayama K., Saito H., and others. Hyperbaric oxygen treatment for multiple sclerosis: short-term and long-term therapy. *Jpn J Hyper Med* 21:215–219, 1986.

27. Davidson D.L.W. Hyperbaric oxygen therapy in the treatment of multiple sclerosis. Report from Action for Research into Multiple Sclerosis, London, England, 1989.

28. Haney D.Q. MS victims find hope in treatment. *The Philadelphia Inquirer* 9/25/83, pp. 1-C, 8-C.

29. Neubauer R.A. Protocol for the treatment of multiple sclerosis with hyperbaric oxygen. *J Hyper Med* 5(1): 53–54, 1990.

Chapter 5
Using HBOT to Treat Difficult Wounds

1. Ehrlich H.P., Grislis G., and Hunt T.K. Metabolic and circulatory contributions to oxygen gradients in wounds. *Surgery* 72:578–583, 1972.

2. Beaman L. and Beaman B.L. The role of oxygen and its derivatives in microbial pathogenesis and host defense. *Ann Rev Microbiol* 38:27–48, 1984.

3. Klebanoff S. Oxygen metabolism and the toxic properties of phagocytes. *Ann Intern Med* 93: 480–489, 1980.

4. Hohn C. Oxygen and leucocyte microbial killing. In Davis J.C. and Hunt T.K. (eds): *Hyperbaric Oxygen Therapy*. Bethesda, Maryland: Undersea Medical Society, 1977, pp. 101–110.

5. Hunt T.K. Disorders of repair and their management. In Hunt T.K. and Dunphy J.E. (eds): *Fundamentals of Wound Management*. New York: Appleton-Century-Crofts, 1979, pp. 68–168.

6. Silver I.A. Cellular microenvironment in healing and non-healing wounds. In Hunt T.K., Heppenstall R.B., Pines E., and others (eds): *Soft and Hard Tissue Repair*. New York: Praeger, 1984, pp. 50–66.

7. Niinikoski J., Hunt T.K., and Zederfeldt B. Oxygen supply in healing tissue. *Am J Surg* 123: 247–252, 1972.

8. Hohn C. Oxygen and leukocyte microbial killing. In Davis J.C. and Hunt T.K. (eds): *Hyperbaric Oxygen Therapy*. Bethesda, Maryland: Undersea and Hyperbaric Medical Society, 1977, pp. 101–110.

9. Hunt T.K. and Pai M.P. The effect of varying ambient oxygen tensions on wound metabolism and collagen synthesis. *Surg Gynecol Obstet* 135:561–567, 1972.

10. Hunt T.K., Niinikoski J., Zederfeldt B.H., and others. Oxygen in wound healing enhancement: cellular effects of oxygen. In Davis J.C. and Hunt T.K. (eds): *Hyperbaric Oxygen Therapy*. Bethesda, Maryland: Undersea Medical Society, 1977, pp. 111–122.

11. Silver I.A. Cellular microenvironment in healing and non-healing wounds. In Hunt T.K., Heppenstall R.B., Pines E., and others (eds): *Soft and Hard Tissue Repair.* New York: Praeger, 1984, pp. 50–66.

12. Knighton D.R., Silver I.A., and Hunt T.K. Regulation of wound healing angiogenesis effect of oxygen gradients and inspired oxygen concentration. *Surgery* 90: 262–270, 1981.

13. Ketchum S.A. III, Thomas A.N., and Hall A.D. Angiographic studies of the effects of hyperbaric oxygen on burn wound revascularization. In Wada J. and Iwa T. (eds): *Proceedings of the Fourth International Congress on Hyperbaric Medicine.* Baltimore: Williams and Wilkins, 1969, pp. 388–394.

14. Wells C.H., Goodpasture J.E., Horrigan D.J., and Hart G.B. Tissue gas measurements during hyperbaric oxygen exposure. In Smith G. (ed): *Proceedings of the Sixth International Congress on Hyperbaric Medicine.* Aberdeen, Scotland: Aberdeen University Press, 1977, pp. 118–124.

15. Strauss M.B. and Hart G.B. Crush injury and the role of hyperbaric oxygen. *Top Emer Med* 6:9–24, 1984.

16. Strauss M.B. and Hart G.B. Compartment syndromes: update and role of hyperbaric oxygen. *HBO Review* 5:163–182, 1984.

17. Sheffield P.J. Tissue oxygen measurements with respect to soft-tissue wound healing with normobaric and hyperbaric oxygen. *HBO Review* 6:18–46, 1985.

18. Strauss M.B., Hargens A.R., Gershuni D.H., Greenberg D.A., Crenshaw A.G., Hart G.B., and Akeson W.H. Reductions of skeletal muscle necrosis using intermittent hyperbaric oxygen in a model compartment syndrome. *J Bone Joint Surg* 65A: 656–662, 1983.

19. Strauss M.B., Hargens A.R., Gershuni D.H., Hart G.B., and Akeson W.H. Delayed use of hyperbaric oxygen for treatment of a model anterior compartment syndrome. *J Ortho Res* 4: 108–111, 1986.

20. Skyhar M.J., Hargens A.R., Strauss M.B., and others. Hyperbaric oxygen reduces edema and necrosis of skeletal muscle in compartment syndromes associated with hemorrhagic hypotension. *J Bone Joint Surg* 68A: 1218–1224, 1986.

21. Nylander G., Lewis D., Nordstrom H., and Larson J. Reduction of postischemic edema with hyperbaric oxygen. *Plast Reconstr Surg* 76:595–603, 1985.

22. Peirce E.C. Pathophysiology, apparatus, and methods including the special techniques of hypothermia and hyperbaric oxygen. In Peirce E.C. (ed): *Extracorporeal Circulation for Open-Heart Surgery.* Springfield, Illinois: Charles C. Thomas, 1969, pp. 83–84.

23. Tan C.M., Im M.J., Myers R.A.M., and others. Effects of hyperbaric oxygen and hyperbaric air on the survival of island skin flaps. *Plast Reconstr Surg* 73:27–30, 1984.

24. Hunt T.K. and van Winkle W. Wound healing: normal repair. In Dunphy J.E. (ed): *Fundamentals of Wound Management in Surgery.* South Plainfield, New

Jersey: Chirurgecom, Inc., 1976, pp. 1–68.

25. Sheffield P.J. Tissue oxygen measurements with respect to soft-tissue wound healing with normobaric and hyperbaric oxygen. *HBO Review* 6:18–46, 1985.

26. Sheffield P.J. Tissue oxygen measurements with respect to soft-tissue wound healing with normobaric and hyperbaric oxygen treatments. In Gottlieb S.F., Longmuir I.S., and Totter J.R. (eds): *Oxygen: An In-Depth Study of Its Pathophysiology.* Bethesda, Maryland: Undersea Medical Society, 1984, pp. 241–277.

27. Kindwall E.P. and Goldmann R.W. *Hyperbaric Medicine Procedures.* Milwaukee, Wisconsin: St. Luke's Hospital, 1984, p. 85.

28. Cianci P. and Bove A. Hyperbaric oxygen therapy in the treatment of acute and chronic peripheral ischemia. *Int Med* 6: 117–137, 1985.

29. Niinikoski J. Effect of oxygen supply on wound healing and formation of experimental granulation tissue. *Acta Physiol Scand* 334:1–72, 1969.

30. Hunt T.K., Conolly W.B., Aronson S.B., and others. Anaerobic metabolism and wound healing: an hypothesis for the initiation and cessation of collagen synthesis in wounds. *Am J Surg* 135:328–332, 1978.

31. Hunt T.K. and Pai M.P. The effect of varying ambient oxygen tensions on wound metabolism and collagen synthesis. *Surg Gynecol Obstet* 135:561–567, 1972.

32. Jones H.P. The role of oxygen and its derivatives in bacterial killing and inflammation. In Gottlieb S.F., Longmuir I.S., and Totter J.R. (eds): *Oxygen: An In-Depth Study of its Pathophysiology.* Bethesda, Maryland: Undersea Medical Society, 1984, pp. 493–516.

33. Hohn D.C. Host resistance of infection: established and emerging concepts. In Hunt T.K. (ed): *Wound Healing and Wound Infection: Theory and Surgical Practice.* New York: Appleton-Century-Crofts, 1980, pp. 264–280.

34. Van Meter K., Lasater S., Whidden S.J., and others. Hyperbaric oxygen therapy and wound healing. *Curr Con Wound Care,* Fall:7–10, 1986.

35. Keck P.E., Gottlieb S.F., and Conley J. Interaction of increased pressures of oxygen and sulfonamides on the *in vitro* and *in vivo* growth of pathogenic bacteria. *Undersea Biomed Res* 7:95–106, 1980.

36. Adams K.R., Sutton T.E., and Mader J.T. *In vitro* potentiation of tobramycin under hyperoxic conditions. *Undersea Biomed Res* 14(suppl):37, 1987.

37. Adams K.R. and Mader J.T. Aminoglycoside potentiation with adjunctive hyperbaric oxygen therapy in experimental *Pseudomonas aeruginosa* osteomyelitis. *Undersea Biomed Res* 14(suppl):37, 1987.

38. Norden C.W. and Kleti E. Experimental osteomyelitis caused by *Pseudomonas aeruginosa. J Infect Dis* 141:71–75, 1980.

39. Hunt T.K., Zederfeldt T.B., and Goldstick T.K. Oxygen and healing. *Am J Surg* 118:521, 1969.

40. Winter G.D. and Perrins

D.J.D. Effects of hyperbaric oxygen treatment on epidermal regeneration. In Wada J. and Iwa T. (eds): *Proceedings of the Fourth International Congress on Hyperbaric Medicine.* Baltimore: Williams and Wilkins, 1969, pp. 363–368.

41. Strauss M.B., Hargens A.R., Gershuni D.H., Hart G.B., and Akeson W.H. Delayed use of hyperbaric oxygen for treatment of a model anterior compartment syndrome. *J Ortho Res* 4: 108–111, 1986.

42. Nylander G., Lewis D., Nordstrom H., and Larson J. Reduction of postischemic edema with hyperbaric oxygen. *Plast Reconstr Surg* 76:595–603, 1985.

43. Kivisaari J. and Niinikoski J. Effects of hyperbaric oxygenation and prolonged hypoxia on the healing of open wounds. *Acta Chirurg Scand* 141:14–19, 1975.

44. Barthelemy L., Bellet M., Michaud A., and Cabon P. The value of thermography in the appreciation of the effectiveness of hyperbaric oxygen therapy in the treatment of acute arteritis of the lower limbs. *Bord Med* 9:1095–1100, 1976.

45. Illingworth C.F., Smith G., Lawson D.D., Ledingham I.M., Sharp G.R., and Griffiths J.C. Surgical and physiological observations in an experimental pressure chamber. *Br J Surg* 49: 222–227, 1961.

46. Loder R.E. Hyperbaric oxygen therapy in acute trauma. *Ann R Coll Surg Engl* 61:472–473, 1979.

47. Maudsley R.H., Hopkinson W.I., and Williams K.G. Vascular injury treated with high pressure oxygen in a mobile chamber. *J Bone Joint Surg* 2(B):346–350, 1963.

48. Schramek A. and Hashmonai M. Vascular injuries in the extremities in battle casualties. *Br J Surg* 64:644–648, 1977.

49. Slack W.K., Thomas D.A., and DeJode L.R.J. Hyperbaric oxygen in the treatment of trauma, ischemia disease of limbs, and varicose ulceration. In: *Proceedings of the Third International Conference on Hyperbaric Medicine.* Publication 1404. Washington: National Academy of Science National Research Council, 1966, pp. 621–624.

50. Szekely O., Szanto G., and Takats A. Hyperbaric oxygen therapy in injured subjects. *Injury* 4:294–300, 1973.

51. Strauss M.B. Role of hyperbaric oxygen therapy in acute ischemias and crush injuries— an orthopedic perspective. *HBO Review* 2:87–106, 1981.

52. Shupak A., Gozal D., Ariel F., Melamed Y., and Katz A. Hyperbaric oxygenation in acute peripheral post-traumatic ischemia. *J Hyper Med* 2:714, 1987.

53. Strauss M.B. and Hart G.B. Hyperbaric oxygen and the skeletal-muscle compartment syndrome. *Contemp Ortho* 18: 167–174, 1989.

54. Strauss M.B. and Hart G.B. Crush injury and the role of hyperbaric oxygen. *Top Emer Med* 6:9–24, 1984.

55. Shupak A., Gozal A.A., and others. Hyperbaric oxygenation in acute peripheral postraumatic ischemia. *J Hyper Med* 2:7–14, 1987.

56. Strauss M.B. and Hart G.B. Hyperbaric oxygen and the

skeletal-muscle compartment syndrome. *Contemp Ortho* 18: 167–174, 1989.

57. Colignon M., Carlier A., Khuc T. and others. Hyperbaric oxygen therapy in acute ischemia and crush injuries. New Horizons in Hyperbaric Medicine Conference, 26–30 April 1989.

58. Monies-Chass I., Maghmonai M., and others. Hyperbaric oxygen treatment as an adjunct to reconstructive vascular surgery in trauma. *Injury* 8:274–277, 1977.

59. Colignon M., Carlier A., Khuc T. and others. Hyperbaric oxygen therapy in acute ischemia and crush injuries. New Horizons in Hyperbaric Medicine Conference, 26–30 April 1989.

Chapter 6
Using HBOT to Treat Infections

1. Gottlieb S.F., Rose N.R., Maurizi J., and Lanphier E.H. Oxygen inhibition of growth of *Mycobacterium* tuberculosis. *J Bacteriol* 87:838–843, 1964.

2. Gottlieb S.F. and Pakman L.M. Effect of high oxygen tensions on the growth of selected, aerobic, gram-negative bacteria. *J Bacteriol* 95:1003–1010, 1968.

3. Gottlieb S.F., Solosky J.A., Aubrey R., and Nedelkoff D.D. Synergistic action of increased oxygen tensions and PABA-folic acid antagonists on bacterial growth. *Aerosp Med* 45:829–833, 1974.

4. Keck P.E., Gottlieb S.F., and Conley J. Interaction of increased pressures of oxygen and sulfonamides on the *in vitro* and *in vivo* growth of pathogenic bacteria. *Undersea Biomed Res* 7:95–106, 1980.

5. Adams K.R., Sutton T.E., and Mader J.T. *In vitro* potentiation of tobramycin under hyperoxic conditions. *Undersea Biomed Res* 14(suppl):37, 1987.

6. Adams K.R. and Mader J.T. Aminoglycoside potentiation with adjunctive hyperbaric oxygen therapy in experimental *Pseudomonas aeruginosa* osteomyelitis. *Undersea Biomed Res* 14(suppl):37, 1987.

7. Norden C.W. and Kleti E. Experimental osteomyelitis caused by *Pseudomonas aeruginosa*. *J Infect Dis* 141:71–75, 1980.

8. Babior B.M. Oxygen-dependent killing by phagoeytes. *New Eng J Med* 298:659–668, 1978.

9. Jones H.P. The role of oxygen and its derivatives in bacterial killing and inflammation. In Gottlieb S.F., Longmuir I.S., and Totter J.R. (eds): *Oxygen: An In-Depth Study of its Pathophysiology*. Bethesda, Maryland: Undersea Medical Society, 1984, pp. 493–516.

10. Hohn D.C. Host resistance of infection: established and emerging concepts. In Hunt T.K. (ed): *Wound Healing and Wound Infection: Theory and Surgical Practice*. New York: Appleton-Century-Crofts, 1980, pp. 264–280.

11. Fischer B., Jain K.K., Braun E., and Lehrl S. *Handbook of Hyperbaric Oxygen Therapy*. Berlin: Springer-Verlag, 1988.

12. Van Unnik A.J.M. Inhibition of toxin production in *Clostridium perfringens* in vitro by hyperbaric oxygen. *Antonie Leeuwenhoek Microbiol* 31:181–186, 1965.

13. Schoemaker G. Oxygen ten-

sion measurements under hyperbaric conditions. In Boerema I., Brummelkamp W.H., and Meijne N.G. (eds): *Clinical Applications of Hyperbaric Oxygen. Proceedings of the First International Congress on Hyperbaric Oxygen.* Amsterdam: Elsevier, 1964, pp. 330–335.

14. Kivisaari J. and Niinikoski J. Use of silastic tube and capillary sampling technique in the measurement of tissue PO^2 and PCO^2. *Am J Surg* 125:623–627, 1973.

15. Sheffield P.J. Tissue oxygen measurements. In Davis J.C. and Hunt T.K. (eds): *Problem Wounds: The Role of Oxygen.* New York: Elsevier, 1988, pp. 17–51.

16. Demello F.J., Hashimoto T., Hitchcock C.R., and Haglin J.J. The effect of hyperbaric oxygen on the germination and toxin production of *Clostridium perfringens* spores. In Wada J. and Iwa J.T. (eds): *Proceedings of the Fourth International Congress on Hyperbaric Medicine.* Baltimore: The Williams & Wilkins Co., 1970, p. 276.

17. Demello F.J., Haglin J.J., and Hitchcock C.R. Comparative study of experimental *Clostridium perfringens* infection in dogs treated with antibiotics, surgery, and hyperbaric oxygen. *Surgery* 73:936–941, 1973.

18. Peirce E.C. II. Gas gangrene: a critique of therapy. *Surg Rounds* 7:17–25, 1984.

19. Bakker D.J. Clostridial myonecrosis. In Davis J.C. and Hunt T.K. (eds): *Problem Wounds: The Role of Oxygen.* New York: Elsevier, 1988, pp. 153–172.

20. Ellis M.E. and Mandal B.K. Hyperbaric oxygen treatment: 10 years' experience of a regional infectious disease unit. *J Infect Dis* 6:187–190, 1971.

21. Hart G.B., Lamb R.C., and Strauss M.B. Gas gangrene I. A collective review. II. A 15-year experience with hyperbaric oxygen. *J Trauma* 23:991–1000, 1983.

22. Brummelkamp W.H., Hogendijk J., and Boerema I. Treatment of anaerobic infections (clostridial myonecrosis) by drenching the tissues with oxygen under high atmospheric pressure. *Surgery* 49:299–302, 1961.

23. Austin F. Maintenance of infective *Borrelia burgdorferi Sh-2-82* in four percent oxygen/five percent carbon dioxide *in vitro*. *Cardio J of Microbiol* 39(12):1103–1110, 1993.

24. Burgdorfer W. National Institutes of Health, Rocky Mountain Laboratory. Personal letter, 10 September 1996.

25. Schwan T. National Institutes of Health, Rocky Mountain Laboratory. Personal letter, 21 August 1996.

26. Fife W.P. and Freeman D.M. Preliminary Clinical Study on the Use of Hyperbaric Oxygen Therapy for the Treatment of Lyme Disease. College Station, Texas: Texas A&M University Hyperbaric Laboratory, 1997 (submitted for publication).

27. Ozorio de Almeida A. and Costa H.M. Treatment of leprosy by oxygen at high pressure associated with methylene blue. *Revist de Leprologia* 6:237–265, 1938.

28. Duenas F.C. Die fruhdiagnose,

therapie und forschung in der lerabekamfung. [The diagnosis, therapy, and investigation of leprosy.] *Das Offentliche Gesundheitswese* 12:667–671, 1969.

29. Wilkinson F.F., Rosasco S.A., Calori B.A., Equia O.F., and Rubio R.A. Conclusions preliminares sobre el uso del oxygeno hiperbaro en lepr lepromatosa. [Preliminary conclusions on the use of hyperbaric oxygen in leprosy.] *Revist de Leprologia* 7: 459–471, 1970.

30. Manheim S.D., Voleti C., Ludwig, A., and Jacobson J.H. Hyperbaric oxygen in the treatment of actinomycosis. *JAMA* 210(3):552–553, 1969.

Chapter 7
Using HBOT to Treat Burns
1. Miller T.A. and Korn H.N. Epithelial burn injury and repair. In Davis J.C. and Hunt T.K. (eds): *Hyperbaric Oxygen Therapy*. Bethesda, Maryland: Undersea Medical Society, 1977, pp. 251–257.

2. Wada J., Ikeda T., Kamada K., and others. Oxygen hyperbaric treatment for severe CO poisoning and severe burns in coal mines (Hokutan-Yubari) gas explosion. *Igaku Jpn* 54:68, 1965.

3. Grossman A.R. Hyperbaric oxygen in the treatment of burns. *Ann Plast Surg* 1/2:163–171, 1978.

4. Wells C.H. and Hilton J.G. Effects of hyperbaric oxygenation on host burn plasma extravasation. In Davis J.C. and Hunt T.K. (eds): *Hyperbaric Oxygen Therapy*. Bethesda, Maryland: Undersea Medical Society, 1977, pp. 259–265.

5. Ketchum S.A., Thomas A.N.,

and Hall A.D. Angiographic studies of the effect of hyperbaric oxygenation on burn wound revascularization. In Wada J. and Iwa T. (eds): *Hyperbaric Medicine*. Baltimore: Williams and Wilkins, 1969, pp. 388–394.

6. Ketchum S.A., Zubrin J.R., Thomas A.N., and others. Effect of HBO on small first, second, and third degree burns. *Surg Forum* 18:65–67, 1967.

7. Arzinger-Jonasch H., Sandner K., and Bittner H. Die widkung hyperbaren sauerstoffs auf brandwunden unterschiedlicher tiefe im tierexperiment. [The effect of hyperbaric oxygen on burn wounds of different depths in animal experiments.] *Z Exp Chir Transplant Kunstliche Organe* 11:6–10, 1978.

8. Kaiser W., Berger A., Leith H., and Heymann H. Hyperbaric oxygenation in burns. *Handchir Mikrochir Plast Chir* 17:326–330, 1985.

9. Hart G.B., O'Reilly R.R., Broussard N.D., and others. Treatment of burns with hyperbaric oxygen. *Surg Gynecol Obstet* 139: 693–696, 1974.

10. Grossman A.R. Hyperbaric oxygen in the treatment of burns. *Ann Plast Surg* 1/2:163–171, 1978.

Chapter 8
Using HBOT to Treat Bone Disorders
1. Harrelson J.M. and Hills B.A. Changes in bone marrow pressure in response to hyperbaric exposure. *Aerosp Med* 41:1018–1021, 1970.

2. Niinikoski J. and Hunt T.K.

Oxygen tensions in healing bone. *Surg Gynecol Obstet* 134: 746–750, 1972.

3. Hunt T.K., Zederfeldt B., and Goldstick T.K. Oxygen and healing. *Am J Surg* 118:521–525, 1969.

4. Strauss M.B. Refractory osteomyelitis. *J Hyper Med* 2:147–159, 1987.

5. Hamblin D.L. Hyperbaric oxygen: its effect on experimental staphylococcal osteomyelitis in rats. *J Bone Joint Surg* 50:1129–1141, 1968.

6. Davis J.C. and Hunt T.K. Refractory osteomyelitis of the extremities and the axial skeleton. In Davis J.C. and Hunt T.K. (eds): *Hyperbaric Oxygen Therapy*. Bethesda, Maryland: Undersea Medical Society, 1977, pp. 217–227.

7. Davis J.C., Heckman J.D., Delee J.C., and Buckwold F.J. Chronic non-hematogenous osteomyelitis treated with adjuvant hyperbaric oxygen. *J Bone Joint Surg* 68:1210–1217, 1986.

8. Morrey B.F., Dunn J.M., Heimbach R.D., and Davis J. Hyperbaric oxygen and chronic osteomyelitis. *Clin Orthop* 144:121–127, 1979.

9. Mainous E.G., Boyne P.J., and Hart G.B. Hyperbaric oxygen treatment of mandibular osteomyelitis: Report of three cases. *J Am Dent Assoc* 87:1426–1430, 1973.

10. Evans B.E., Jacobson J.H., Peirce E.C., Friedman E.W., and Schwartz A.E. Chronic osteomyelitis of mandible. *NY State J Med* 76(6):966–967, 1976.

11. Walder D.N. Aseptic necrosis in bone. In Strauss R.H. (ed): *Diving Medicine*. New York: Grune and Stratton, 1976, pp. 97–108.

12. Bonfiglio M. Development of bone necrosis lesions. In Lambertsen C.J. (ed): *Underwater Physiology V. Proceedings of the Fifth Symposium on Underwater Physiology*. Bethesda, Maryland: Federation of American Societies for Experimental Biology, 1976, pp. 117–132.

13. Jones J.P. Jr. Osteonecrosis. In McCarty D.J. (ed): *Arthritis and Allied Conditions: A Textbook of Rheumatology*. Philadelphia: Lea and Febiger, 1979, pp. 1121–1134.

14. Laufer A. Aseptic necrosis of the femoral head. *J Mt Sinai Hosp* 24:957–987, 1957.

15. Black K.A., Khangure M.S., and Owen E.T. Dexamethasone and osteonecrosis. *Aust NZ J Med* 11:521–525, 1981.

16. Neubauer R.A., Kagan R.L., and Gottlieb S.F. Use of hyperbaric oxygen for the treatment of aseptic bone necrosis: a case study. *J Hyper Med* 4:69–76, 1989.

17. Neubauer R.A., Kagan R.L., and Gottlieb S.F. Use of hyperbaric oxygen for the treatment of aseptic bone necrosis: a case study. *J Hyper Med* 4:69–76, 1989.

18. Neubauer R.A., Kagan R.L., and Gottlieb S.F. Use of hyperbaric oxygen for the treatment of aseptic bone necrosis: a case study. *J Hyper Med* 4:69–76, 1989.

19. Conti V., Tassy J., Leonardelli M., and Ohresser P. Limits of hyperbaric oxygen in the treatment of aseptic bone necrosis in the femoral head. *Bull Med Sub Hyp* 1:3–4, 1969.

20. Sainty J.M., Conti V., Aubert L., and Allessandrini G. Role of hyperbaric oxygen in the treatment of aseptic bone necrosis of the hip. *Med Aeronaut Spat Med Subaquatique Hyperbare* 19: 215–217, 1980.

21. Baixe J.H., Bidart J., and Nicolini J.C. Treatment of osteonecrosis of the femoral head by hyperbaric oxygen. *Bull Med Sub Hyp* 1:2, 1969.

22. Mainous E.G. Osteogenesis enhancement utilizing hyperbaric oxygen therapy. *HBO Review* 3:181–185, 1982.

23. Mainous E.G., Boyne P.J., and Hart G.B. Hyperbaric oxygen treatment of mandibular osteomyelitis: Report of three cases. *J Am Dent Assn* 87: 1426–1430, 1973.

24. Strauss M.B., Malluche H.H., and Faugere M.C. Effect of hyperbaric oxygen on bone resorption in rabbits. Seventh Annual Conference on Clinical Application of HBO, Anaheim, California, 8–18 June 1982.

25. Mainous E.G. Osteogenesis enhancement utilizing hyperbaric oxygen therapy. *HBO Review* 3:181–185, 1982.

26. Davis J.C. and Hunt T.K. Refractory osteomyelitis of the extremities and axial skeleton. In Davis J.C. and Hunt T.K. (eds): *Hyperbaric Oxygen Therapy.* Bethesda, Maryland: Undersea Medical Society, 1977, pp. 217–227.

27. Kulagin L.M., Varguzina V.I., Kirsanove L.N., and others. Regenerative potentials of tissue under HBO conditions depending on the character of the injury. In Yefuni S.N. (ed): *Abstracts of the Seventh International Congress of HBO Medicine,* Moscow: USSR Academy of Sciences, 1981, pp. 326–327.

28. Tikhilow R.M., Akimov G.C., and Lotovin A.P. Effects of oxygen barotherapy on the regeneration of bone tissue. *Orthop Traumatol Protez* 12:51–52, 1980.

29. Sepnov V.N. and Uglova M.V. Features of sternum regeneration in autoplasty under conditions of hyperbaric oxygen. *Orthop Traumatol Protex* 5:51–53, 1979.

30. Zavesa P.X., Shavab Y.Y., and Abduchudonov S.S. Effects of local oxygen therapy on reparative regeneration of the bone. *Orthop Traumatol Protez* 1:71–72, 1977.

31. Neubauer R.A. and Maxfield J.R. Nonunion fracture treated 33 months after injury with hyperbaric oxygen. *Med Subacquea ed Iperbarica Minerva Med* 1:23–26, 1984.

Chapter 9
Using HBOT to Treat Complications of Radiation Treatment and Skin Surgery

1. Heimbach R.D. Radiation effect on tissues. In Davis J.C. and Hunt T.K. (eds): *Problem Wounds: The Role of Oxygen.* New York: Elsevier, 1988, pp. 53–63.

2. Mainous E.G. Hyperbaric oxygen in maxillofacial osteomyelitis, osteoradionecrosis, and osteogenesis enhancement. In Davis J.C. and Hunt T.K. (eds): *Hyperbaric Oxygen Therapy.* Bethesda, Maryland: Undersea Medical Society, 1977, pp. 191–203.

3. Greenwood T.W. and Gilchrist

A.G. Hyperbaric oxygen and wound healing in post-irradiation head and neck surgery. *Br J Surg* 50:394, 1973.

4. Hart G.B. and Strauss M.B. Hyperbaric oxygen in the management of radiation injury. In Schmutz J. (ed): *Proceedings of the First Swiss Symposium on Hyperbaric Medicine.* Basel, Switzerland: Foundation for Hyperbaric Medicine, 1986, pp. 31–51.

5. Boden G. Radiation myelitis of the cervical spinal cord. *Br J Radiol* 21:464, 1948.

6. Luk K.H., Baker D.G., and Fellows C.F. Hyperbaric oxygen after radiation and its effect on the production of radiation myelitis. *Int J Radiat Oncol Bio Phys* 4:457–459, 1978.

7. Hopewell J.W. Hyperbaric oxygenation after irradiation and its effect on the production of radiation myelitis. *Int J Radiat Oncol Bio Phys* 5:1917, 1979.

8. Torubarov F.S., Pakhomov V.I., Krylova I.V., and others. Changes in cerebral hemodynamics in patients with vascular pathology in the late stages of radiation sickness treated with hyperbaric oxygenation. *Zh Neuropatol Psikhiatr* 83:28–33, 1983.

9. Hart G.B. and Strauss M.B. Hyperbaric oxygen in the management of radiation injury. In Schmutz J. (ed): *Proceedings of the First Swiss Symposium on Hyperbaric Medicine.* Basel, Switzerland: Foundation for Hyperbaric Medicine, 1986, pp. 31–51.

10. Ferguson B.J., Hudson W.R., and Farmer J.C. Hyperbaric oxygen therapy for laryngeal radionecrosis. *Ann Otol Rhinol Laryngol* 96:1–6, 1987.

11. Hart G.B. and Strauss M.B. Hyperbaric oxygen in the management of radiation injury. In Schmutz J. (ed): *Proceedings of the First Swiss Symposium on Hyperbaric Medicine.* Basel, Switzerland: Foundation for Hyperbaric Medicine, 1986, pp. 31–51.

12. Bakker D.J. and Rijkmans B.G. Hyperbaric oxygen in the treatment of radiation-induced hemorrhagic cystitis: a report on 10 cases. In Schmutz J. and Bakker D. (eds): *Proceedings of the Second Swiss Symposium on Hyperbaric Medicine.* Basel, Switzerland: Foundation for Hyperbaric Medicine, 1989.

13. Hart G.B. and Strauss M.B. Hyperbaric oxygen in the management of radiation injury. In Schmutz J. (ed): *Proceedings of the First Swiss Symposium on Hyperbaric Medicine.* Basel, Switzerland: Foundation for Hyperbaric Medicine, 1986, pp. 31–51.

14. Weiss J.P. and Neville E.C. Hyperbaric oxygen: primary treatment of radiation-induced hemorrhagic cystitis. *J Urol* 142:43–45, 1989.

15. Hart G.B. and Strauss M.B. Hyperbaric oxygen in the management of radiation injury. In Schmutz J. (ed): *Proceedings of the First Swiss Symposium on Hyperbaric Medicine.* Basel, Switzerland: Foundation for Hyperbaric Medicine, 1986, pp. 31–51.

16. Glassburn J.R., Brady L.W., and Plenk H.P. Hyperbaric oxygen in radiation therapy. *Cancer* 39:751–765, 1977.

17. Hart G.B. and Strauss M.B. Hyperbaric oxygen in the management of radiation injury. In Schmutz J. (ed): *Proceedings of the First Swiss Symposium on Hy-*

perbaric Medicine. Basel, Switzerland: Foundation for Hyperbaric Medicine, 1986, pp. 31–51.

18. Kindwall E.P. and Goldman R.W. *Hyperbaric Medicine Procedures*. Milwaukee, Wisconsin: St. Luke's Hospital, 1988.

19. Hart G.B. and Strauss M.B. Hyperbaric oxygen in the management of radiation injury. In Schmutz J. (ed): *Proceedings of the First Swiss Symposium on Hyperbaric Medicine*. Basel, Switzerland: Foundation for Hyperbaric Medicine, 1986, pp. 31–51.

20. Marx R.E., Johnson R.P., and Kline S.N. Prevention of osteoradionecrosis: a randomized prospective clinical trial of hyperbaric oxygen versus penicillin. *J Am Dent Assn* 111:49–54, 1985.

21. Kaufman T., Hirshowitz B., and Monies-Chass I. Hyperbaric oxygen for postirradiation osteomyelitis of the chest wall. *Harefuah* 97:220–222, 271, 1979.

22. Hart G.B. and Strauss M.B. Hyperbaric oxygen in the management of radiation injury. In Schmutz J. (ed): *Proceedings of the First Swiss Symposium on Hyperbaric Medicine*. Basel, Switzerland: Foundation for Hyperbaric Medicine, 1986, pp. 31–51.

23. Hart G.B. and Strauss M.B. Hyperbaric oxygen in the management of radiation injury. In Schmutz J. (ed): *Proceedings of the First Swiss Symposium on Hyperbaric Medicine*. Basel, Switzerland: Foundation for Hyperbaric Medicine, 1986, pp. 31–51.

24. Marx R.E. and Johnson R.P. Problem wounds in oral and maxillofacial surgery: the role of hyperbaric oxygen. In Davis J.C. and Hunt T.K. (eds): *Problem Wounds: The Role of Oxygen*. New York: Elsevier, 1988, pp. 65–123.

25. Champion W.M., McSherry C.K., and Goulian, D. Effect of hyperbaric oxygen on the survival of the pedicled skin flaps. *J Surg Res* 7(12), 1967.

26. Boerema I. An operating room for high oxygen pressure. *Surgery* 47:291–298, 1961.

27. Perrins J.D. Hyperbaric oxygenation of ischemic skin flaps and pedicles. In Brown I.W. and Cox B.G. (eds): *Proceedings of the Third International Congress on HBO Medicine*. Durham, North Carolina: Duke University Press, 1966, pp. 613–620.

28. Perrins J.D. Influence of hyperbaric oxygen on the survival of split skin grafts. *Lancet* 1: 868–871, 1967.

29. Perrins J.D. Influence of hyperbaric oxygen on the survival of split skin grafts. In Wada J. and Iwa T. (eds): *Proceedings of the Fourth International Congress on HBO Medicine*. London: Baillere, 1970, pp. 369–376.

30. Shulman A.G. and Krohn H.L. Influence of hyperbaric oxygen and multiple skin allographs on the healing of skin wounds. *Surgery* 62(6):1051–1058, 1967.

31. Wilmeth J.B. and Gazaui A. Hyperbaric oxygen as an adjunct to the treatment of orthopedic injuries with full thickness grafts. Seventh Annual Conference on the Clinical Application of HBO, Anaheim, California, 9–11 June 1982.

32. Bass B.H. The treatment of varicose leg ulcers by hyperbaric oxygen. *Postgrad Med J* 46:407–408, 1970.

33. Fisher B.H. Hyperbaric oxy-

gen for skin ulcers. *Roche Med Image Commentary*, 1969.

34. Olejniczak S. Employment of low hyperbaric therapy in management of leg ulcers. *Mich Med,* 1969.

35. Rosenthal A.M. Treatment of patients with pressure sores in the hyperbaric chamber. *Proceedings of the American Congress of Rehabilitation in Medicine.* New York, 1970.

Chapter 10
Using HBOT to Treat Posioning

1. Chance B., Erecinska M., and Wagner M. Mitochondrial responses to carbon monoxide toxicity. *Ann NY Acad Sci* 174: 193–204, 1970.

2. Marklund S.L. Oxygen toxicity and protective systems. *Clin Toxicol* 23:289–298, 1985.

3. Coburn R.F. Mechanisms of carbon monoxide toxicity. *Pre Med* 8:310–322, 1979.

4. Halebian P., Robinson N., Barie P., Goodwin C., and Shires G.T. Whole body oxygen utilization during acute carbon monoxide poisoning and isocapnic nitrogen hypoxia. *J Trauma* 26:110–117, 1986.

5. Walum E., Varnbo I., and Peterson A. Effects of dissolved carbon monoxide on the respiratory activity of perfused neuronal and muscle cell cultures. *Clin Toxicol* 23: 299–308, 1985.

6. Raybourn M.S., Cork C., Schimmerling W., and Tobins C.A. An *in vitro* electrophysiological assessment of the direct cellular toxicity of carbon monoxide. *Toxicol Appl Pharmacol* 46:769–779, 1978.

7. Ingenito A.J. and Durlacher L. Effects of carbon monoxide on the beta wave of the cat electroretinogram: comparisons with nitrogen hypoxia, epinephrine, vasodilator drugs and changes in respiratory tidal volume. *J Pharmacol Exp Ther* 211: 636–646, 1979.

8. Goldbaum L.R., Ramirez R.G., and Absalon K.B. What is the mechanism of carbon monoxide toxicity? *Aerosp Med* 46:1289–1291, 1975.

9. Haldane J.S. The relation of action of carbonic oxide to oxygen tension. *J Physiol (London)* 18:201–217, 1895.

10. End E. and Long C.W. HBO in carbon monoxide poisoning. I. Effect on dogs and guinea pigs. *J Ind Hyg Toxicol* 24:302–306, 1942.

11. Valois J.D. and Schade J.P. An electrophysiological study of histotoxic anoxia under normal and hyperbaric conditions. In Bour H. and Ledingham I.M.C. (eds): *Carbon Monoxide Poisoning.* New York: Elsevier, 1967, pp. 183–197.

12. Araki R., Nashimoto I., and Takano T. The effect of hyperbaric oxygen on cerebral hemoglobin oxygenation and dissociation rate of carboxyhemoglobin in anesthetized rats: spectroscopic approach. *Adv Exp Med Biol* 222:375–381, 1988.

13. Smith G., Ledingham I.M., Sharp G.R., and others. Treatment of coal-gas poisoning with oxygen at 2 atmospheres of pressure. *Lancet* 1:816–818, 1962.

14. Ziser A., Shupak A., Halpern P., and others. Delayed hyperbaric oxygen treatment for acute carbon monoxide poison-

ing. *BMJ* 289:960, 1984.

15. Neubauer R.A. Carbon monoxide and hyperbaric oxygen. *JAMA* 139:629, 1979.

16. Winter A. and Shatin L. Hyperbaric oxygen in reversing carbon monoxide coma. *NY State J Med* 70:889–894, 1970.

17. Welsh F., Matos L., and DeTreville R.T.P. Medical hyperbaric oxygen therapy. *Aviat Space Environ Med* 51:611–614, 1980.

18. Yee L.M. and Brandon G.K. Successful reversal of presumed carbon monoxide-induced semicoma. *Aviat Space Environ Med* 54:641–643, 1983.

19. Rioux J.P. and Myers R.A.M. Hyperbaric oxygen for methylene chloride poisoning. *Ann Emer Med* 18:691–695, 1989.

20. Yacoub M.H. and Zeitlin G.L. Hyperbaric oxygen in the treatment of postoperative low output cardiac syndrome. *Lancet* i:581–583, 1965.

21. Cabalane M. and Demling R.H. Early respiratory abnormalities from smoke inhalation. *JAMA* 251:771–773, 1984.

22. Takashi H., Kobayashi S., and Sakakibara K. The value of hyperbaric oxygen therapy in preventing late manifestations following acute carbon monoxide poisoning. In Kindwall, E.P. (ed): *Proceedings of the Eighth International Congress on Hyperbaric Medicine.* San Pedro, California: Best, 1987, pp. 274–281.

23. Thom S.R. Smoke inhalation. *Emer Clin North Am* 7: 371–387, 1989.

24. Myers R.A.M., Snyder S.K., Emhoff T.A., and others. Subacute sequelae of carbon monoxide poisoning. *Ann Emer Med* 14:1163–1167, 1985.

25. Lacey D.J. Neurologic sequelae of acute carbon monoxide intoxication. *Am J Dis Child* 135: 145, 1981.

26. Binder J.W. Carbon monoxide intoxication in children. *Clin Toxicol* 16:287, 1980.

27. Goxal D., Ziser A., Shupak A., and others. Accidental carbon monoxide poisoning. *Clin Ped* 24:132–135, 1985.

28. Raphael J.C., Elkharrat D., Jars-Giuncestre M.C., and others. Trial of normobaric and hyperbaric oxygen for acute carbon monoxide intoxication. *Lancet* ii:414–419, 1989.

29. Ducasse J.L., Izard P.H., Celsis P., and others. Moderate carbon monoxide poisoning: hyperbaric or normobaric oxygenation? Human randomized study with tomographic cerebral blood flow measurement. In Schmutz J. and Bakker D. (eds): *Proceedings of the Second Swiss Symposium on Hyperbaric Medicine.* Basle, Switzerland: Foundation for Hyperbaric Medicine, 1988.

30. Thom S.R. Experimental carbon monoxide-mediated brain lipid peroxidation and the effects of oxygen therapy. *Ann Emer Med* 17:403, 1988.

31. Trapp W.G. and Lepawsky M. 100% survival in five life-threatening acute cyanide poisoning victims treated by a therapeutic spectrum including hyperbaric oxygen. First European Congress Hyperbaric Medicine, Amsterdam, 7–9 September 1983.

32. Kindwall E.P. and Goldmann R.W. *Hyperbaric Medicine Procedures.* Milwaukee, Wisconsin: St. Luke's Hospital, 1988.

33. Bitterman N., Talmi Y., and Lerman E. The effects of hyperbaric oxygen on acute experimental sulfide poisoning in the rat. *Toxicol Appl Pharmacol* 84:325–328, 1986.

34. Smilkstein M.J., Bronstein A.C., Pickett H.M., and others. Hyperbaric oxygen therapy for severe hydrogen sulfide poisoning. *J Emer Med* 3:27–30, 1985.

35. Whitecraft D.D., Bailey T.D., and Hart G.B. Hydrogen sulfide poisoning treated with hyperbaric oxygen. *J Emer Med* 3:23–25, 1985.

36. Hsu P., Lo H.W., and Line Y.T. Acute hydrogen sulfide poisoning treated with hyperbaric oxygen. *J Hyper Med* 2:212–221, 1987.

37. Saltzman H.A. Acute hepatic injury due to carbon tetrachloride poisoning and use of hyperbaric oxygen therapy. *HBO Review* 2:171–174, 1981.

38. Troop B.R., Majerus T., Bernacchi A., and others. Hyperbaric oxygen improves survival in rats poisoned with carbon tetrachloride. *J Hyper Med* 1:157–161, 1986.

39. Montana S. and Perret C. HBO during experimental intoxication with carbon tetrachloride. *Rev Fr Etud Clin Biol* 12:274–278, 1967.

40. Truss C.D. and Killenberg P.G. Treatment of carbon tetrachloride poisoning with hyperbaric oxygen. *Gastroenterology* 82:767–769, 1982.

41. Saltzman H.A. Acute hepatic injury due to carbon tetrachloride poisoning and use of hyperbaric oxygen therapy. *HBO Review* 2:171–174, 1981.

42. Larcan V., Laprevote-Heully M.C., Lambert H., and others. Intoxication and ingestion of a massive dose of carbon tetrachloride. Recovery probably related to early hyperbaric oxygen therapy. *Ann Chir* 28: 445–454, 1973.

43. Smith R.P. and Olson M.V. Drug induced methemoglobinemia. *Semin Hematol* 10:253–268, 1973.

44. Sheehy M.H. and Way J.L. Nitrite intoxication: protection with methylene blue and oxygen. *Toxicol Appl Pharmacol* 30: 221–226, 1974.

Chapter 11
Using HBOT to Treat Circulatory Problems

1. Dawber T.R. *The Framingham Study.* Boston: Harvard University Press, 1980, pp. 62–75.

2. Dinkel R., Bochner K., and Pampuro M. *Socio-economic importance of vein disorders.* Health Econ. LTD, Health Service Consultants, Basle, Switzerland. Nineth World Congress of Phlebology, Kyoto, Japan, 22–26 September 1986.

3. Dinkel R., Bochner K., and Pampuro M. *Socio-economic importance of vein disorders.* Health Econ. LTD, Health Service Consultants, Basle, Switzerland. Nineth World Congress of Phlebology, Kyoto, Japan, 22–26 September 1986.

4. Fruhling L. and Baltzenschlager A. Anatomie pathologie de l'arteriosclerose. [Anatomy of the pathology of arteriosclerosis.] In: *Rapport au 33 Congres Francais de Medecine.* Paris: Masson, 1961, pp. 97–142.

5. Cloarec M. Correlations entre

les differentes localisations arte'rielles coronaires, gastro-intestinalse et peripheriques de l'atherosclerose. [Correlations of different locations of atherosclerosis in aterioles in the heart, gastro-intestinal system, and peripherally.] In Sandoz (ed): *Rapport au 4th Congres du College Francais de pathologie Vasculaire.* Paris, 1970.

6. Cristol R. *Las Aspects Polyarteriels de L'arterosclerose.* [The Aspects of Arteriosclerosis in Many Arteries.] Vol. 1. Paris: Slyvoxyl-Wander, 1972.

7. Dawber T.R. *The Framingham Study.* Boston: Harvard University Press, 1980, pp. 62–75.

8. Hertzer N.R., Beven E.G., Young J.R., and O'Hara P.J. Incidental asymptomatic carotid bruits in patients scheduled for peripheral vascular reconstruction: results of cerebral and coronary angiography. *Surgery* 535–543, 1984.

9. Mitchel J. and Schewartz C. Relationship between arterial disease in different sites. A study of the aorta and coronary carotid and iliac arteries. *Br J Med* 1:1293–1301, 1962.

10. Bloor K. Natural history of arteriosclerosis of the lower extremities. *Ann R Coll Surg Engl* 28:36–52, 1961.

11. Jeurgens J.L., Barker N.W., and Hines G.A. Arteriosclerosis obliterans: review of 250 cases with special references to pathogenic and prognostic factors. *Circulation* 41:875–883, 1960.

12. Bloor K. Natural history of arteriosclerosis of the lower extremities. *Ann R Coll Surg Engl* 28:36–52, 1961.

13. Nielsen J. Arteriosclerosis obliterans of the lower extremities in nondiabetic men: survival and causes of death. *Dan Med Bull* 10–17, 1975.

14. Dawber T.R. *The Framingham Study.* Boston: Harvard University Press, 1980, pp. 62–75.

15. Kannel W.B. and Shurtless B. The natural history of arterlosclerosis obliterans. *Cardiovasc Clin* 3:37–52, 1971.

16. Jain K.K. Hyperbaric oxygen therapy in cardiovascular diseases. In Jain K.K. (ed): *Textbook of Hyperbaric Medicine.* Toronto: Hogrefe & Huber, 1990, p. 334.

17. Jain K.K. Hyperbaric oxygen therapy in cardiovascular diseases. In Jain K.K. (ed): *Textbook of Hyperbaric Medicine.* Toronto: Hogrefe & Huber, 1990, pp. 334–335.

18. Fredenucci P. Oygenotherapie hyperbare en patholgie vasculaire. 19 annees d'expeience. [Nineteen years of experience with hyperbaric oxygenation and vascular pathology.] IXth Congress of European Undersea Biomedical Society, Barcelona, September 1983.

19. Fredenucci P. Arteriopathies et O.H.B. *Medecine du Dud-Est* 6300–6306, 1982.

20. Kindwall E.P. *Hyperbaric Medicine Procedures.* Milwaukee, Wisconsin: St. Luke's Hospital, 1979, p. 17.

21. Yefuni S.N., Lyskin G.I., and Fokina T.S. Hyperbaric oxygenation in treatment of peripheral vascular disorders. *Int Angiol* 4:207–209, 1985.

22. Fischer B. and Wein Den Hammer W. Selsbstbeurteilungsskala fur leichte formen der zerebralen insuffizienz. [Self-review scale for light forms of

cerebral insufficiency.] In Lehrl S. and others (eds): *Diagnose und Therapiekontrolle von organisetten Psychosyndromen.* Vless, Holland: Ehensberg, 1972.

23. Dormandy J.A., Hoare E., Colley J., Arrowsmith D.E., and Dormandy T.L. Clinical haemodynamic, rheological, and biochemical findings in 126 patients with intermittent claudications. *BMJ* 4:576, 1973.

24. Di Perri T. Rheological factors in circulatory disorders. *Angiology* 30:480, 1979.

25. Bird A.D. and Telfer A.B.M. Effect of hyperbaric oxygen on limb circulation. *Lancet* 13:355–356, 1965.

26. Stalker C.G. and Ledingham I.M.A. The effect of increased oxygen in prolonged acute limb ischemia. *Br J Surg* 60:959–963, 1973.

27 Mottram R.F. Effects of hyperbaric oxygen on limb circulation. *Lancet* 13:602, 1965.

28. Ackerman N.B. and Brinkley F.B. Oxygen tensions in normal and ischemic tissues during hyperbaric therapy. *JAMA* 198:142–145, 1966.

29. Kawamura M., Sakakibara K., and Yusa T. Effect of increased oxygen on peripheral circulation in acute, temporary limb hypoxia. *J Cardiovasc* 19:161–168, 1978.

30. Schraibman I.G., Ledingham F.R.C.S., and Ledingham, I.M.A. Hyperbaric oxygen and regional vasodilation in pedal ischemia. *Surg Gynecol Obstet* 125: 761–767, 1969.

31. Nylander G., Lewis H., Nordstrom H., and Larsson J. Reduction of postischemic edema with hyperbaric oxygen. *Plast Reconstr Surg* 76:602–603, 1985.

32. Illingworth C.F.W. Treatment of arterial occlusion under oxygen at two atmospheres absolute. *BMJ* 2:1272, 1962.

33. Fredenucci P. Oxygenotherapie hyperbarre et arteriopathies. [Hyperbaric oxygen in the treatment of arteriopathologies.] *J Mal Vasc* 10(Suppl A):166–172, 1985.

34. Gerard R., Fredenucci P., Barthelemy L., Bourde J., Lamy J., Jouve A., and Appaix A. L'oxygene hyperbare dans le traitement des arteriopathies. [Hyperbaric oxygen in the treatment of arteriopathologies.] *Arch Mal Coeur* 4:472–483; 1967.

35. Kostiunin V.N., Pahkomov V.I., Feoktistov P.L., and others. Increasing the effectiveness of hyperbaric oxygenation in the treatment of patients with stage IV arterial occlusive disease of the lower limbs. *Vestn Khir* 135: 48–51, 1985.

36. Baroni G., Porro T., Fuglia E., and others. Hyperbaric oxygen in diabetic gangrene treatment. *Diabetes Care* 10:81–86, 1987.

37. Belov K.V., Isakov Y.V., and Alyabaiev V.S. Efficacy of hyperbaric oxygenation on the activity of succinated hydrogenase and cytochrome oxidase of visceral organs in intestinal obstruction. *Anesteziol Reanimatol* 5: 44–46, 1986.

38. Urayama H., Takemura H., Kasaima F., and others. Hyperbaric oxygen therapy for chronic occlusive disease of the extremities. *Nippon Geka Gakkai Zasshi* 993:429–433, 1992.

39. Kovacevic H. The investigation of hyperbaric oxygen influence in the patients with sec-

ond degree of atherosclerotic insufficiency of lower extremities. Ph.D. diss., University of Rieka, Croatia, 1992.

40. Jain K.K. Hyperbaric oxygen therapy in cardiovascular diseases. In Jain K.K. (ed): *Textbook of Hyperbaric Medicine.* Toronto: Hogrefe & Huber, 1990, pp. 338–340.

Huber, 1995, pp. 446–463.

4. Reillo M. *AIDS Under Pressure.* Kirkland, Washington: Hogrefe & Huber, 1997, pp. 51–53.

5. Reillo M. *AIDS Under Pressure.* Kirkland, Washington: Hogrefe & Huber, 1997, pp. 39–45.

6. Reillo M. *AIDS Under Pressure.* Kirkland, Washington: Hogrefe & Huber, 1997, pp. 39–45.

Chapter 12
Using HBOT to Treat AIDS

1. Jain K.K. *Textbook of Hyperbaric Medicine.* Toronto: Hogrefe & Huber, 1995, pp. 317–341.
2. Williams S. The social stigma and health risks of Kaposi's sarcoma are giving way to a treatment revolution. *Poz,* August 1997, pp. 72–85.
3. Jain K.K. *Textbook of Hyperbaric Medicine.* Toronto: Hogrefe &

Conclusion

1. Kolata G. Flawed treatment of head injuries found. *The New York Times,* 16 October 1991, p. C14.
2. Ruiz E., Brunette D.D., Robinson E.P., and others. Cerebral resuscitation after cardiac arrest using hetasterch hemodilution, hyperbaric oxygenation, and magnesium ion. *Resuscitation* 14:213–223, 1986.

GLOSSARY

Italicized words are defined elsewhere in the glossary.

ABN. See *aseptic bone necrosis.*

Acoustic trauma. Ear damage that can occur after a sudden, sharp noise, such as an explosion or a gunshot.

Acquired immune deficiency syndrome (AIDS). A condition in which the immune system is destroyed, leaving the patient vulnerable to *opportunistic infection*. It is caused by infection with the human immunodeficiency virus (HIV) and cofactor herpes viruses.

Actinomycosis ("lumpy jaw"). An infection that causes deep, lumpy holes which produce pus.

Aerobic organisms. Microbes that thrive in the presence of oxygen. *Hyperbaric oxygen therapy* may be able to counteract these microbes indirectly by stimulating the immune system.

Age-related macular degeneration (AMD). A wasting of either the optic nerve or the macula, the spot on the retina within the eye where vision is most acute.

AIDS. See *acquired immune deficiency syndrome.*

Air embolism. The development of air bubbles within the bloodstream caused by tears in the lungs. This can happen to a diver who ascends to the surface while holding his or her breath. Air emboli usually migrate to the brain, and are often fatal.

AMD. See *age-related macular degeneration.*

Anaerobic organisms. Microbes that can grow in the absence of oxygen. *Hyperbaric oxygen therapy* can both counteract the reproduction of these microbes and neutralize their lethal toxins.

Angina pectoris. Acute chest pain caused by spasms that squeeze the coronary arteries. These spasms reduce blood flow to the heart, and thus reduce the heart's oxygen supply.

Angioplasty. An operation used to relieve *peripheral vascular disease* and coronary artery disease. A tube is placed in a clotted blood vessel, and the clot is then either flattened with a tiny balloon or destroyed with a laser.

Arteriosclerosis obliterans. A condition in which fatty deposits form on the walls of the peripheral arteries. It is a form of *peripheral vascular disease.*

Aseptic bone necrosis (ABN). A painful bone inflammation caused by reduced blood flow within the bone. It most often occurs among divers as a consequence of *decompression sickness,* but can also occur spontaneously or as a complication of disease.

ATA. See *atmospheres absolute.*

Atherosclerosis. The buildup of fatty deposits in the arteries. This condition can lead to *heart attack* or *stroke* if the affected artery becomes completely blocked. It can also cause *peripheral vascular disease.*

Atmospheres absolute (ATA). The unit of pressure measurement used in *hyperbaric oxygen therapy.* One atmospheres absolute is the average atmospheric pressure exerted at sea level.

Bends, the. See *decompression sickness.*

Blood-brain barrier. A protective layer of cells that keeps many types of toxins from reaching the brain.

Buerger's disease. A condition in which the arteries in the legs become clotted and inflamed.

Cerebral hemorrhage. Bleeding within the brain, leading to a *stroke.*

Cerebrospinal fluid. The fluid that surrounds the brain and spinal cord.

Coma. A state of deep unconsciousness in which the patient does not respond to external stimulation.

Compartment syndrome. A condition in which inward pressure on an artery leads to a reduction in blood flow and consequent *hypoxia.*

Coronary-artery disease. A condition in which the arteries that bring blood to the heart become blocked. It can lead to a *heart attack.*

Cyanosis. A blueness of the skin and mucous membranes produced by *hypoxia.*

Decompression sickness ("the bends"). A serious condition in which gas bubbles escape into the bloodstream. It is generally caused by a diver ascending too quickly.

Difficult wound. A wound in which *hypoxia* leads to disruption of the wounded area's blood supply, which in turn makes the wound slow to heal.

Dormant neurons ("idling neurons"). Brain cells within the *penumbra* that have been stunned but not damaged by a *stroke* or other brain injury.

Edema. A swelling of the tissues, such as that caused by injury or *stroke*.

EEG. See *electroencephalogram*.

Electroencephalogram (EEG). A test used to record brain waves. It is used in cases of *stroke* or other brain injury.

Embolic (thrombotic) occlusion. A condition in which a small piece of fat or a blood clot becomes stuck in a blood vessel, blocking the flow of blood to a limb. It is a form of *peripheral vascular disease*.

Endarterectomy. An operation used to relieve *peripheral vascular disease* in which clotted material is removed from a blood vessel.

Fracture nonunion. A bone fracture that fails to heal.

Free radical. A molecule that can cause tissue damage when involved in an uncontrolled chemical reaction. Free radicals are produced both by normal bodily processes and by abnormal conditions.

Gas gangrene. A painful infection that causes swelling, massive tissue death, and gas production. It can be fatal if not treated quickly.

Hansen's disease. See *leprosy*.

HBOT. See *hyperbaric oxygen therapy*.

Heart attack. A condition in which an artery leading to the heart is blocked off, resulting in the development of an *infarct* in the heart muscle.

Heart failure. A condition in which the heart is unable to pump blood efficiently to all parts of the body, resulting in *edema* and breathing difficulties.

Hemoglobin. The substance in *red blood cells* that binds with oxygen and carries it throughout the body. Poisons such as carbon monoxide bind with hemoglobin instead of oxygen, causing oxygen shortages within the tissues.

Hyperbaric oxygen therapy (HBOT). The use of oxygen at greater-than-normal-*atmospheric* pressure to force oxygen into the body's tissues and thus promote healing.

Hyperbaricist. A doctor or other health care professional who is trained to administer *hyperbaric oxygen therapy*.

Hypoxia. Underoxygenation of the body's tissues.

Idling neurons. See *dormant neurons*.

Infarct. An area of decayed tissue caused by a lack of oxygen, resulting in tissue death. Both *strokes* and *heart attacks* can cause infarcts.

Intermittent claudication. A condition in which leg cramps occur after walking. It is caused by *peripheral vascular disease.*

Ischemia. A lack of blood flow caused by narrowing or blockage of an artery. It can be caused by *atherosclerosis*.

Ischemic cascade. The first phase of a *stroke*. In this phase, which doctors believe lasts from between two minutes and four to six hours, the lack of blood and oxygen triggers a cycle of ever-increasing damage.

Kaposi's sarcoma. A viral infection that causes both purplish skin lesions and lesions within the body. It is an *opportunistic infection* associated with *acquired immune deficiency syndrome*.

Lacuna. A small hole within the brain caused by the withering of an *infarct*.

Leprosy (Hansen's disease). A chronic bacterial disease that can cause disfigurement and loss of sensation.

Lumpy jaw. See *actinomycosis*.

Lyme disease. A tickborne illness that can bring about nerve, heart, and joint problems if not treated promptly. Initial symptoms include a bull's-eye rash.

MAC. See *mycobacterium avium complex*.

Methemoglobinemia. A condition in which *red blood cells* cannot carry a full amount of oxygen because their *hemoglobin* has been damaged. A variety of toxic substances can produce this condition.

Microcirculation. The flow of blood through the capillaries, the tiny blood vessels that connect arteries to veins. Microcirculation is often disrupted by *hypoxia*.

Migraine headache. An especially severe headache preceded by sensory disturbances and associated with nausea and vomiting. It is caused by changes in blood flow to the brain, and occurs on only one side of the head.

Monoplace chamber. A hyperbaric oxygen chamber that holds one person.

MS. See *multiple sclerosis.*

Multiplace chamber. A hyperbaric oxygen chamber that holds two or more people.

Multiple sclerosis (MS). A condition in which nerve fibers in the brain and spinal cord lose their protective covering, and thus do not properly transmit nerve impulses. It is responsible for sight disturbances, weakness and paralysis, abnormal reflexes, and slurred speech.

***Mycobacterium avium* complex (MAC).** A bacterial infection that causes fever, diarrhea, and abdominal pain. It is an *opportunistic infection* associated with *acquired immune deficiency syndrome.*

Omentum transposition. An operation in which an abdominal membrane called the omentum is tailored and brought, under the skin, to a damaged area in the brain or spinal cord. The membrane provides a rich supply of blood vessels and growth factors.

Opportunistic infection. An infection that generally affects people with damaged immune systems. A number of these infections, including *Kaposi's sarcoma, Pneumocystis carinii pneumonia,* and *Mycobacterium avium complex,* are associated with *acquired immune deficiency syndrome.*

Osteomyelitis. A bone infection that can develop after injury or surgery, or can travel to the bone from elsewhere in the body. It may cause pain, swelling, and fever.

PCP. See *pneumocystis carinii pneumonia.*

Penumbra. The area between brain tissue damaged by a *stroke* or other brain injury and the surrounding healthy tissue. The penumbra contains *dormant neurons* that can be stimulated by *hyperbaric oxygen therapy.*

Peripheral vascular disease (PVD). Disease that occurs in blood vessels other than such major vessels as the aorta.

Physiological transection. An event that sometimes follows severe spinal cord bruises, in which swelling, lack of oxygen, and production of toxins all combine to prevent nerve impulses from passing through the transected area.

Plaques. Hardened, scarred patches in the brain and spinal cord that often develop as the result of *multiple sclerosis.*

Plasma. The liquid portion of the blood.

Plasticity. The ability of the brain to reorganize itself after a *stroke* or other brain injury. Plasticity allows healthy areas of the brain to take over functions normally performed by areas that have been damaged.

***Pneumocystis carinii* pneumonia (PCP).** A form of pneumonia that generally affects both lungs. It is an *opportunistic infection* associated with *acquired immune deficiency syndrome.*

Port wine stain. An often unsightly birthmark caused by excess blood vessels in the skin.

Problem wound. See *difficult wound.*

PVD. See *peripheral vascular disease.*

Radionecrosis. Tissue damage caused by radiation treatment.

Raynaud's disease. A condition in which blood flow to the extremities is interrupted. It can cause coldness, numbness, tingling, and pain.

Red blood cells. The blood cells that contain *hemoglobin*, which carries oxygen throughout the body.

Single photon emission computerized tomography (SPECT). A body-imaging system that uses a radioactive tracer to show the location of active brain cells. It is a useful tool in following the progress of *stroke* and brain-injured patients who are undergoing *hyperbaric oxygen therapy*.

Skin grafting. A procedure in which healthy skin taken from the patient's own body is used to cover a wound or burn. It is often used in cosmetic surgery.

Spasticity. Rigidity of the muscles. It is a common after-effect of *stroke* or other brain injury.

SPECT. See *single photon emission computerized tomography*.

Stasis dermatitis. A condition in which reduced circulation to the legs results in swollen ankles and skin problems.

Stroke. A condition in which a reduction of blood flow to or within the brain leads to the development of an *infarct*. The symptoms produced depend on what area of the brain is affected.

Sympathectomy. An operation used to relieve *peripheral vascular disease*. A nerve, usually located in the upper thigh, is cut. This can cause tightened blood vessels to relax.

TIA. See *transient ischemic attack*.

Tinnitus. A buzzing, hissing, or ringing sound in the ears.

Tissue plasminogen activator (TPA). A drug that breaks

up blood clots. It is used in cases of *heart attack* and certain kinds of *stroke.*

TPA. See *tissue plasminogen activator.*

Transient ischemic attack (TIA). A temporary *stroke*-like condition in which blood flow is reduced to a localized area of the brain. The occurrence of a TIA can be a warning signal of a major stroke in the future. By definition, a TIA will heal spontaneously within twenty-four hours with no residual damage.

Traumatic arterial occlusion. A condition in which an injured artery interferes with blood flow to a limb. It is a form of *peripheral vascular disease.*

Vasodilators. Drugs that dilate the blood vessels.

Vein bypass or replacement. An operation used to relieve *peripheral vascular disease.* A diseased section of vein is either bypassed or replaced, with either a synthetic vein or a vein taken from elsewhere in the patient's body.

White blood cells. The blood cells that fight infection.

Index